新时代高等院校大学英语系列教材

专门用途英语系列

总主编 俞洪亮

医学英语读写教程

Medical English Reading and Writing

主 编 王 燕 熊淋宵 罗海鹏

副主编（按姓氏音序）
褚宏蕊 汪 媛 张 洁

编 委（按姓氏音序）
董 俭 顾兼美 黎 丽 李冠颖 李怡然
宋晓慧 王 燕 熊淋宵 袁 琳

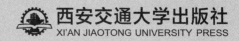

西安交通大学出版社
XI'AN JIAOTONG UNIVERSITY PRESS

图书在版编目(CIP)数据

医学英语读写教程 / 王燕，熊淋宵，罗海鹏主编. —
西安 ：西安交通大学出版社，2023.7
新时代高等院校大学英语系列教材 / 俞洪亮总主编
ISBN 978 - 7 - 5693 - 3169 - 1

Ⅰ.①医… Ⅱ.①王… ②熊… ③罗… Ⅲ.①医学-
英语-阅读教学-高等学校-教材 ②医学-英语-写作-
高等学校-教材 Ⅳ. ①R

中国国家版本馆 CIP 数据核字(2023)第 062775 号

书　　　名	医学英语读写教程	
主　　　编	王　燕　熊淋宵　罗海鹏	
总 主 编	俞洪亮	
责任编辑	庞钧颖	
责任校对	牛瑞鑫	

出版发行	西安交通大学出版社
	(西安市兴庆南路 1 号　邮政编码 710048)
网　　址	http://www.xjtupress.com
电　　话	(029)82668357　82667874(市场营销中心)
	(029)82668315(总编办)
传　　真	(029)82668280
印　　刷	陕西天意印务有限责任公司

开　　本	889mm×1194mm　1/16　印张 11　字数 318 千字
版次印次	2023 年 7 月第 1 版　　2023 年 7 月第 1 次印刷
书　　号	ISBN 978 - 7 - 5693 - 3169 - 1
定　　价	49.00 元

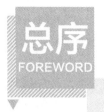

总序
FOREWORD

当今世界正处在百年未有之大变局,以新能源、新材料、大数据、人工智能等为代表的新一轮科技革命加速演进。中国制造 2025、教育现代化 2035 等国家重大战略布局,对高等教育发展尤其是人才培养和人才供给产生了深刻的影响,也提出了全新的命题。我们要把准新一轮科技革命和产业革命的脉搏,坚持以社会需求为导向,深入推进本科专业布局调整和教育教学改革,让一流本科教育真正满足新时代对一流本科人才的需求。

世界现代大学发展史表明,本科教育是高等教育的立命之本、发展之本。回归本科教育已经成为世界一流大学共同的行动纲领。党和国家加快推动本科教育振兴,持续推进本科人才培养模式改革,从"四新建设"到"双万计划",从构建高校思政工作体系到全面实施课程思政……推进一流本科教育的步伐行稳致远、张弛有度。2019 年 9 月,教育部印发《关于深化本科教育教学改革 全面提高人才培养质量的意见》,同年 12 月,教育部印发《普通高等学校教材管理办法》,对立德树人的人才培养根本任务、课程建设质量的全面提高和高水平教材的编写及使用等方面提出了意见。

发展外语教育是全球的共识,外语教育伴随国家发展阶段的变化而变化。进入新时代,外语教育的使命与责任更加重大,高等外语教育的发展关系到高等教育人才的培养质量。在中国新一轮的高等教育改革中,大学英语教育教学要立足新的发展阶段,主动服务国家战略需求,主动融入新文科建设,适应高等教育普及化阶段的需求和特点,拥抱新未来和新技术,在建设更高质量的课程中获取改革与发展的新动能,在融合发展中开辟大学英语课程建设的新路径。

教材关乎国家事权,是铸魂工程,是构建高质量高等教育体系的重要内容,也是课堂教学的重要载体和实现人才培养的有力保障。因此,推进新时代教材建设,必须体现马克思主义中国化要求,体现中国和中华民族风格,体现党和国家对教育的基本要求,体现国家和民族基本价值观,体现人类文化知识积累和创新成果。2021 年是中国共产党成立 100 周年和"十四五"规划开局之年,也是开启全面建设社会主义现代化国家新征程的第一年,我们在这个重要历史节点上,以全面贯彻党的教育方针,落实立德树人根本任务为宗旨,紧扣国家对推进新文科建设的需求,并以《大学英语教学指南(2020 版)》为指导,组织编写了这套"新时代高等院校大学英语系列"教材,力求培养心系祖国发展、积极参与全球竞争、思维方式创新、融贯中西文化的新时代人才。

本系列教材分为两个子系列,分别为"大学通识教育课程系列"和"专门用途英语系列",以知识、能力、素养和价值为本位,体现通识教育与专业教育的有机结合。具体来讲,本系列教材的特色如下。

1. 思政统领,落实立德树人的根本任务,坚持价值和能力双重导向

"新时代高等院校大学英语系列"教材全面贯彻党的教育方针,落实立德树人根本任务,扎根中国大地,站稳中国立场,充分体现社会主义核心价值观,强化爱国主义、集体主义、社会主义教育,展现中华优秀传统文化,将构建人类命运共同体、"一带一路"倡议、中国制造2025等热点话题有机融入教材编写,使学生在真实场景中习得知识,提升能力,引导学生坚定道路自信、理论自信、制度自信、文化自信,增强学生"讲好中国故事"的底气和能力。

2. 聚焦一流建设,融入"双万计划",发挥示范引领作用

本系列教材遵循高起点、高标准、高要求的原则,融入一流专业和一流课程建设,对标金课"两性一度",反映学科发展的最新进展,引入高等外语教育改革最新成果。我们力求从体系搭建、内容架构、问题设置等方面打造全方位、多维度的示范性教材。

3. 融入"四新"建设,体现学科交叉融合,服务创新人才体系

大学英语教育在新工科、新医科、新农科和新文科建设中被赋予了新的责任和使命。面对新一轮的科技浪潮和全球变局,大学英语教育成为创新型、复合型、应用型、国际化人才培养体系的重要一环,也是服务跨学科创新人才培养的不可或缺的基础。本系列教材中不仅有对人工智能、大数据和区块链发展等新兴交叉学科的探讨,也有对医学、艺术、教育、科技、农业等传统领域的拓展。这些教材能够帮助不同学科背景的学生拓宽视野,培养创新思维,增强思辨能力。

4. 坚持"学生中心"育人理念,尊重个体差异,实现教学资源多样化

智能教育时代学生的思维特点、学习习惯和现代信息技术的持续发展都对教材的内容和形态提出了新的要求。学生学习的方式和获取资源的渠道日趋多样化,教材也要走好线上线下融合的道路。同时,教师的教育观、教学观、教材观、学生观、质量观等均发生了变化。多形态的教材建设和数字化学习资源供给成为新一轮大学英语建设的重要内容。本系列教材配套慕课、示范微课、在线练习、音频和视频等各类知识服务资源,产生"教"与"学"的互动,提升学生的参与感、获得感和成就感。

5. 面向中西部高校,推动优质教育均衡发展,满足学生更高水平的需求

高等教育的整体质量是我国构建高质量教育体系的重要影响因素。本系列教材加强东部与西部高校间协同合作,观照中西部地区高等院校目标读者,增加展现中西部地区人文特色以及社会和科技发展成果的最新内容,依据中西部高校的教学实际编写,适应国家和区域经济社会发展需求。

"新时代高等院校大学英语系列"教材编写团队成员均是具有丰富教学经验、专业知识背景和先进教学理念的骨干教师,来自西安交通大学、兰州大学、西北工业大学、西安电子科技大学、扬州大学、西北师范大学、宁夏大学、河南科技大学、西安外国语大学、西北政法大学等多所院校。

一流人才培养须"知行合一"。我们组织编写的这套具有中西部特色,体现东部与西部合作的高水平、高质量、高起点的"新时代高等院校大学英语系列"教材正是对国家人才培养战略部署的积极响应,希望它如同一艘航船,带领老师和同学们驶向更广阔的海洋。

在国家"一带一路"倡议和高等学校"双一流"建设背景下,高校医学专业领域的国际研究和合作交流项目越来越多,中国医疗队积极参与国际医疗救助和人道主义救助,为世界医疗卫生事业贡献中国力量。新时代下的国际医疗人才,不仅要有扎实的医学知识,还应通晓医学专业英语。

医学英语是专门用途英语的一个分支。随着我国医学科学的迅速发展,医学英语的重要性日益突显,在临床工作、医学研究和国际医学学术交流活动中发挥着不可或缺的作用。医学英语也是影响医务工作者专业发展的重要因素。不仅如此,新时代还对医学教育提出了新要求。2020 年,《国务院办公厅关于加快医学教育创新发展的指导意见》明确提出要"全力提升院校医学人才培养质量","培养医德高尚、医术精湛的人民健康守护者"。因此,高校医学英语课程的教学也应体现课程思政。医学英语课程的选材不但要注重对医学英语知识和技能的培养,还要兼顾医学人文素养的熏陶。

《医学英语读写教程》在立足医学英语教学实际的基础上,引入先进的教学理念,采用科学的教学设计和丰富的练习活动,以提高学生医学英语应用能力,提升教师课堂教学质量,助力医学人才培养。该教材在设计和编写中采用医文结合的方式来编排内容,每个单元既包括人体系统的基础知识与常见疾病的临床知识,又选编了权威期刊中常见疾病的相关叙事作品,体现了医学知识与人文素养的有机结合。教材还遵循"以教师为主导、以学生为主体"的教学理念,在设计练习活动时,借鉴基于使用的语言学习观等国内外先进的二语习得理论,采用任务式、项目式、合作式等教学方法,帮助学生高效学习医学英语。

该教材的编写团队根据多年医学英语教学经验,精心选材,重点培养学生的医学英语阅读能力、写作能力与叙事医学能力。教材内容可读性强、练习活动丰富、内容设计科学,配有课件及阅读材料的来源,有利于提升学生自主学习能力,便于教学活动的开展。总之,《医学英语读写教程》是一本注重知识性、凸显实用性、体现时代性的教材,能够满足高等医学院校本科生的教学需求。

白永权教授

随着新医科建设的推进,医学教育不断改革,以提升医学人才培养质量。大学英语教育是医学教育的重要组成部分。《大学英语教学指南(2020版)》明确要求大学英语课程应落实立德树人的根本任务,面向医学生的医学英语课程也应体现课程思政。目前,大多数医学英语教材侧重医学英语知识和技能的讲解,较少兼顾医学人文素养。在此背景下,《医学英语读写教程》应运而生。

编写思路

《医学英语读写教程》编写团队认真贯彻《中国教育现代化2035》和《国务院办公厅关于加快医学教育创新发展的指导意见》等文件精神,在编写中严格遵循以下原则。

❖ 教学内容:医文融合

《医学英语读写教程》按照人体系统编排,每个单元包括人体系统的基础知识、常见疾病的临床知识及相关叙事作品,将医学知识与人文素养有机结合。常见疾病的选择依据最新发表于国际权威医学期刊《柳叶刀》的中国疾病负担研究报告;叙事作品主要为医生、患者以及患者家属撰写的医学故事,语言地道、情感真实。医文融合的教学内容设计方式,有助于学生在提升语言技能的同时巩固医学知识、塑造高尚医德。

❖ 教学目标:能力导向

《医学英语读写教程》的整体教学目标是培养学生医学英语阅读能力、写作能力和叙事医学能力,为医学生的临床工作和医学研究奠定英语语言基础。围绕整体目标,每个单元的学习目标按照单元内容及学习难度而设定。

❖ 教学理念:学生为主

《医学英语读写教程》在教学目标、教学内容与练习活动的设计上充分考虑学生的自主性,激发学生的自主学习兴趣,培养学生的自主学习能力。

❖ 练习活动:科学有效

在设计练习活动时,《医学英语读写教程》以国内外先进的二语习得理论为指导,采用任务式、项目式、合作式等教学方法,帮助学生高效学习医学英语。

教材特色

本教材的特色主要体现在如下方面。

❖ 选材可读性强

考虑到选材内容和语言难度过大可能会影响学生学习的积极性,教材中选取的阅读材料难度适中、可读性强。医学知识部分的文章具有准确性与科学性,人文故事的选材具有思辨性与趣味性,让学生在提高英语水平的同时,巩固医学知识,传承医学精神。

❖ 练习丰富多样

教材中的练习活动形式多样,包括图形标注、完形填空、回答问题、思维导图、句子排序、书面描述、仿写句子、读后续写、小组讨论、项目汇报等,从词汇、句子、段落、语篇等不同层面培养学生的医学英语应用能力。

❖ 设计科学合理

教材的每个单元由 Learning objectives、Theme reading 1、Vocabulary bridge、Theme reading 2、Story sharing 和 Vocabulary checklist 这 6 个部分构成。每单元学习目标(Learning objectives)清晰明确,循序渐进。Theme reading 1 介绍人体系统的基础知识。Theme reading 2 介绍常见疾病的临床知识。Vocabulary bridge 通过对常见疾病、症状及体征的解释将两篇主题阅读相连接。Story sharing 涉及 Theme reading 2 中的疾病,从人文角度引发学生对临床诊疗、临终关怀等问题的深度思考。Vocabulary checklist 主要以单词和词组方式列出与本单元主题相关的英文表达,同时标出高频医学英语词汇,方便学生学习。

❖ 教学资源立体

教材配有课件及相关学习材料的出处,便于教师和学生自行查找、学习及使用。

教学建议

《医学英语读写教程》为基础级别的医学英语读写教材,适合临床医学、预防医学、麻醉学、儿科学、医学影像学、医学检验技术等专业的本科生。对于大学英语六级以下水平的学习者,建议学习 64 学时;对于大学英语六级及以上水平的学习者,建议学习 32 学时。

编写分工

《医学英语读写教程》的编写团队由 6 所医学院校的 13 位医学英语教师组成。滨州医学院的王燕(第一章)、黎丽(第二章)、宋晓慧(第六章)和袁琳(第七章),以及北京中医药大学的李怡然(第三章)、李冠颖(第四章)、熊淋宵(第五章)和董俭(第八章)这 8 位老师主要负责教材的编写;江苏联合职业技术学院南通卫生分院的罗海鹏老师和顾兼美老师、济宁医学院的褚宏蕊老师、南京医科大学的张洁老师和安徽医科大学的汪媛老师主要负责教材的审核。

《医学英语读写教程》的出版得到了滨州医学院、北京中医药大学及江苏联合职业技术学院南通卫生分院的大力支持;西安交通大学出版社对教材的定稿和出版给予了宝贵的建议,深表感谢。

由于编者水平与经验有限,书中难免有不妥之处,恳请读者批评指正。

编　者

2022 年 12 月 6 日

目录
CONTENTS

Chapter 1　Cardiovascular system ·································· (1)

Learning objectives ·· (1)

Theme reading 1　**An introduction to the cardiovascular system** ······ (1)

Vocabulary bridge ·· (6)

Theme reading 2　**Stroke** ··· (7)

Story sharing ·· (14)

Vocabulary checklist ·· (17)

Chapter 2　Respiratory system ································· (22)

Learning objectives ·· (22)

Theme reading 1　**An introduction to the respiratory system** ············ (22)

Vocabulary bridge ·· (27)

Theme reading 2　**Lung cancer** ······································· (27)

Story sharing ·· (34)

Vocabulary checklist ·· (36)

Chapter 3　Digestive system ··································· (42)

Learning objectives ·· (42)

Theme reading 1　**An introduction to the digestive system** ············· (42)

Vocabulary bridge ·· (47)

Theme reading 2　**Liver cancer** ······································· (48)

Story sharing ·· (55)

Vocabulary checklist ·· (59)

Chapter 4　Urinary system ····································· (65)

Learning objectives ·· (65)

Theme reading 1　**An introduction to the urinary tract** ··············· (65)

Vocabulary bridge ·· (69)

Theme reading 2　**Chronic kidney disease** ····························· (70)

Story sharing ·· (76)

Vocabulary checklist ·· (79)

Chapter 5　Reproductive system ······························· (82)

Learning objectives ·· (82)

Theme reading 1　**An introduction to the reproductive system** ········· (82)

Vocabulary bridge ·· (89)

Theme reading 2　**Ovarian cancer** ·· (90)

Story sharing ·· (95)

Vocabulary checklist ·· (98)

Chapter 6　Endocrine system ·· (103)

Learning objectives ·· (103)

Theme reading 1　**An introduction to the endocrine system** ············· (103)

Vocabulary bridge ·· (108)

Theme reading 2　**Diabetes** ·· (109)

Story sharing ·· (115)

Vocabulary checklist ·· (118)

Chapter 7　Nervous system ·· (124)

Learning objectives ·· (124)

Theme reading 1　**An introduction to the nervous system** ··············· (124)

Vocabulary bridge ·· (129)

Theme reading 2　**Alzheimer's disease** ······································ (129)

Story sharing ·· (137)

Vocabulary checklist ·· (141)

Chapter 8　Musculoskeletal system ·· (146)

Learning objectives ·· (146)

Theme reading 1　**An introduction to the musculoskeletal system** ············· (146)

Vocabulary bridge ·· (152)

Theme reading 2　**Arthritis** ·· (153)

Story sharing ·· (158)

Vocabulary checklist ·· (161)

Cardiovascular system

Upon completion of this chapter, you will be able to
∴ name the parts of the heart and the vessels that carry blood to and from it;
∴ describe blood circulation;
∴ list major pathologic conditions affecting the heart and blood vessels;
∴ understand information about stroke;
∴ gather information about common cardiovascular diseases;
∴ present one common cardiovascular disease with group members.

Theme reading 1

An introduction to the cardiovascular system[①]

What does the heart do?

The heart is a pump, usually beating about 60 to 100 times per minute. With each heartbeat, the heart sends blood throughout our bodies, carrying oxygen to every cell. After delivering the oxygen, the blood returns to the heart. The heart then sends the blood to the lungs to pick up more oxygen. This cycle repeats over and over again.

What does the cardiovascular system do?

The cardiovascular system is made up of heart and blood vessels that carry blood away from and towards the heart. Arteries carry blood away from the heart and veins carry blood back to the heart.

The cardiovascular system carries oxygen, nutrients, and hormones to cells, and removes waste products, like carbon dioxide. These roadways travel in one direction only, to keep

---

① Adapted from "Heart and circulatory system." Hirsch, L. (2018). https://kidshealth.org

things going where they should.

What are the parts of the heart?

The heart has four chambers—two on top and two on bottom. The two bottom chambers are the right ventricle and the left ventricle. These pump blood out of the heart. A wall called the interventricular septum is between the two ventricles. The two top chambers are the right atrium and the left atrium. They receive the blood entering the heart. A wall called the interatrial septum is between the atria.

The atria are separated from the ventricles by the atrioventricular valves. The tricuspid valve separates the right atrium from the right ventricle. The mitral valve separates the left atrium from the left ventricle.

Two valves also separate the ventricles from the large blood vessels that carry blood leaving the heart. The pulmonic valve is between the right ventricle and the pulmonary artery, which carries blood to the lungs. The aortic valve is between the left ventricle and the aorta, which carries blood to the body.

What are pathways of blood circulation?

Two pathways come from the heart. The pulmonary circulation is a short loop from the heart to the lungs and back again. The systemic circulation carries blood from the heart to all the other parts of the body and back again.

The pulmonary artery is a big artery that comes from the heart. It splits into two main branches, and brings blood from the heart to the lungs. At the lungs, the blood picks up oxygen and drops off carbon dioxide. The blood then returns to the heart through the pulmonary veins.

Next, blood that returns to the heart has picked up lots of oxygen from the lungs. So it can now go out to the body. The aorta is a big artery that leaves the heart carrying this oxygenated blood. Branches of the aorta send blood to the muscles of the heart itself, as well as all other parts of the body. Like a tree, the branches get smaller and smaller as they get farther from the aorta.

At each body part, a network of tiny blood vessels called capillaries connects the very small artery branches to very small veins. The capillaries have very thin walls, and through them, nutrients and oxygen are delivered to the cells. Waste products are brought into the capillaries.

Capillaries then lead into small veins. Small veins lead to larger and larger veins as the blood approaches the heart. Valves in the veins keep blood flowing in the correct direction. Two large veins that lead into the heart are the superior vena cava and inferior vena cava. (The terms superior and inferior don't mean that one vein is better than the other, but that they're located above and below the heart.)

Once the blood is back in the heart, it needs to re-enter the pulmonary circulation and go back to the lungs to drop off the carbon dioxide and pick up more oxygen.

How does the heart beat?

The heart gets messages from the body that tell it when to pump more or less blood depending on a person's needs. For example, when you're sleeping, it pumps just enough to provide for the lower amounts of oxygen needed by your body at rest. But when you're exercising, the heart pumps faster so that your muscles get more oxygen and can work harder.

How the heart beats is controlled by a system of electrical signals in the heart. The sinus (or sinoatrial) node is a small area of tissue in the wall of the right atrium. It sends out an electrical signal to start the contracting (pumping) of the heart muscle. This node is called the pacemaker of the heart because it sets the rate of the heartbeat and causes the rest of the heart to contract in its rhythm.

These electrical impulses make the atria contract first. Then the impulses travel down to the atrioventricular (or AV) node, which acts as a kind of relay station. From here, the electrical signal travels through the right and left ventricles, making them contract.

One complete heartbeat is made up of two phases. The first phase is called systole. This is when the ventricles contract and pump blood into the aorta and pulmonary artery. During systole, the atrioventricular valves close, creating the first sound (the lub) of a heartbeat. When the atrioventricular valves close, it keeps the blood from going back up into the atria. During this time, the aortic and pulmonary valves are open to allow blood into the aorta and pulmonary artery. When the ventricles finish contracting, the aortic and pulmonary valves close to prevent blood from flowing back into the ventricles. These valves closing is what creates the second sound (the dub) of a heartbeat. The second phase is called diastole. This is when the atrioventricular valves open and the ventricles relax. This allows the ventricles to fill with blood from the atria, and get ready for the next heartbeat.

How can I keep my heart healthy?

To help keep your heart healthy, you could get plenty of exercise, eat a nutritious diet, reach and keep a healthy weight, quit smoking if you smoke, go for regular medical checkups, and tell the doctor about any family history of heart problems.

Let the doctor know if you have any chest pain, trouble breathing, or dizzy or fainting spells; or if you feel like your heart sometimes goes really fast or skips a beat.

(1,052 words)

Task 1

Read the passage above and answer the following questions.

(1) What does the heart do?

(2) What does the cardiovascular system do?

(3) What are the parts of the heart?

(4) What are pathways of blood circulation?

(5) How does the heart beat?

(6) What can you do to keep your heart healthy?

Task 2

Please label Figure 1-1 with the medical terms you have learnt in Theme reading 1.

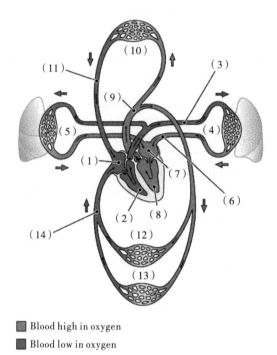

Blood high in oxygen

Blood low in oxygen

Figure 1-1　The cardiovascular system[①]

(1)	(2)
(3)	(4)
(5)	(6)
(7)	(8)
(9) aorta	(10) Capillaries of head and arms
(11)	(12) Capillaries of internal organs
(13) Capillaries of legs	(14)

---

① Adapted from *Medical terminology: an illustrated guide* (*7th edition*). Cohen, B. J., & DePetris, A. (2014). Philadelphia: Lippincott Williams & Wilkins.

Task 3

In Figure 1-2, each number represents a step of blood circulation. Please describe each step by one or two sentences and write them down on the blanks below the figure.

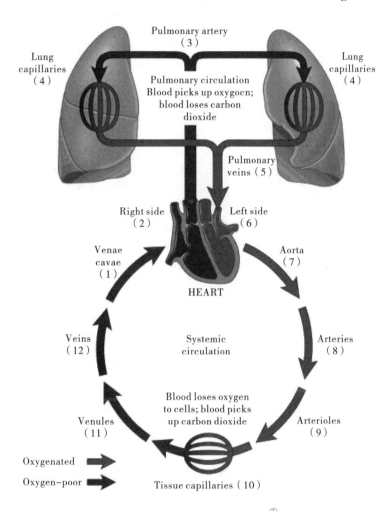

Figure 1-2   Blood circulation[①]

(1)

(2)

(3)

(4)

(5)

①Adapted from *The language of medicine (10th edition)*. Chabner, D-E. (2014). Canada: Saunders.

(6)

(7)

(8)

(9)

(10)

(11)

(12)

Vocabulary bridge

Study the following terms for common signs, symptoms and diseases related to the cardiovascular system and translate them into Chinese.

Medical terms	Explanation	Chinese translations
aneurysm	localized dilation of the wall of a blood vessel, usually an artery, due to a congenital defect or weakness in the vessel wall	动脉瘤
angina pectoris	mild to severe pain or pressure in the chest caused by ischemia; also called angina	
arrythmia	irregularity or loss of rhythm of the heartbeat; also called dysrhythmia	
arteriosclerosis	thickening, hardening, and loss of elasticity of arterial walls; also called hardening of the arteries	
atherosclerosis	most common form of arteriosclerosis, caused by accumulation of fatty substances within the arterial walls, resulting in partial and, eventually, total occlusion	
coronary artery disease (CAD)	abnormal condition that affects the heart's arteries and produces various pathological effects, especially reduced flow of oxygen and nutrients to the myocardium	
deep vein thrombosis (DVT)	formation of a blood clot in a deep vein of the body, occurring most commonly in the iliac and femoral veins	
heart failure (HF)	condition in which the heart cannot pump enough blood to meet the metabolic requirement of body tissues; formerly called congestive heart failure (CHF)	

Medical terms	Explanation	Chinese translations
hypertension	consistently elevated blood pressure that is higher than 119/79 mmHg, causing damage to the blood vessels and, ultimately, the heart	
ischemia	inadequate supply of oxygenated blood to a body part due to an interruption of blood flow	
mitral valve prolapse (MVP)	condition in which the leaflets of the mitral valve prolapse into the left atrium during systole, resulting in incomplete closure and backflow of blood	
murmur	abnormal sound heard on auscultation, caused by defects in the valves or chambers of the heart	
myocardial infarction (MI)	necrosis of a portion of cardiac muscle caused by partial or complete occlusion of one or more coronary arteries; also called heart attack	
rheumatic heart disease	streptococcal infection that causes damage to the heart valves and heart muscle, most commonly in children and young adults	
stroke	damage to part of the brain due to interruption of its blood supply caused by bleeding within brain tissue or, more commonly, blockage of an artery, also called cerebrovascular accident (CVA)	
thrombus	aggregation of platelets, fibrin, clotting factors, and the cellular elements of the blood attached to the interior wall of a vein or artery, sometimes occluding the lumen of the vessel; also called blood clot	
transient ischemic attack (TIA)	temporary interference in the blood supply to the brain that causes no permanent brain damage	
varicose veins	swollen superficial veins that are visible through the skin and usually occur in the legs	

Theme reading 2

Stroke[1]

A stroke, sometimes called a brain attack, occurs when something blocks blood supply to part of the brain or when a blood vessel in the brain bursts. In either case, parts of the brain

---

① Adapted from "About stroke"(n. d.). https://www.cdc.gov

become damaged or die. A stroke can cause lasting brain damage, long-term disability, or even death.

Types of stroke

The type of stroke you have affects your treatment and recovery.

The three types of stroke are ischemic stroke, hemorrhagic stroke and transient ischemic attack (TIA).

Most strokes (87%) are ischemic strokes. An ischemic stroke happens when blood flow through the artery that supplies oxygen-rich blood to the brain becomes blocked. Blood clots often cause the blockages that lead to ischemic strokes.

A hemorrhagic stroke happens when an artery in the brain leaks blood or ruptures (breaks open). The leaked blood puts too much pressure on brain cells, which damages them. High blood pressure and aneurysms—balloon-like bulges in an artery that can stretch and burst—are examples of conditions that can cause a hemorrhagic stroke.

There are two types of hemorrhagic strokes. Intracerebral hemorrhage is the most common type of hemorrhagic stroke. It occurs when an artery in the brain bursts, flooding the surrounding tissue with blood. Subarachnoid hemorrhage is a less common type of hemorrhagic stroke. It refers to bleeding in the area between the brain and the thin tissues that cover it.

A TIA is sometimes called a "mini-stroke." It is different from the major types of stroke because blood flow to the brain is blocked for only a short time—usually no more than 5 minutes.

It is important to know the following points. A TIA is a warning sign of a future stroke. It is a medical emergency, just like a major stroke. Strokes and TIAs require emergency care. Call 120 right away if you feel signs of a stroke or see symptoms in someone around you. There is no way to know in the beginning whether symptoms are from a TIA or from a major type of stroke. Like ischemic strokes, blood clots often cause TIAs. More than a third of people who have a TIA and don't get treatment have a major stroke within 1 year. As many as 10% to 15% of people will have a major stroke within 3 months of a TIA.

Recognizing and treating TIAs can lower the risk of a major stroke. If you have a TIA, your health care team can find the cause and take steps to prevent a major stroke.

Signs and symptoms

During a stroke, every minute counts! Fast treatment can lessen the brain damage that stroke can cause.

By knowing the signs and symptoms of stroke, you can take quick action and perhaps save a life—maybe even your own.

Symptoms of stroke in men and women are

• sudden numbness or weakness in the face, arm, or leg, especially on one side of the body;

- sudden confusion, trouble speaking, or difficulty understanding speech;
- sudden trouble seeing in one or both eyes;
- sudden trouble walking, dizziness, loss of balance, or lack of coordination;
- sudden severe headache with no known cause.

Call 120 right away if you or someone else has any of these symptoms.

Acting F. A. S. T. can help stroke patients get the treatments they desperately need. The stroke treatments that work best are available only if the stroke is recognized and diagnosed within 3 hours of the first symptoms. Stroke patients may not be eligible for these if they don't arrive at the hospital in time.

If you think someone may be having a stroke, act F. A. S. T. and do the following simple test:

F—Face: Ask the person to smile. Does one side of the face droop?

A—Arms: Ask the person to raise both arms. Does one arm drift downward?

S—Speech: Ask the person to repeat a simple phrase. Is the speech slurred or strange?

T—Time: If you see any of these signs, call 120 right away.

Note the time when any symptoms first appear. This information helps health care providers determine the best treatment for each person. Do not drive to the hospital or let someone else drive you. Call an ambulance so that medical personnel can begin life-saving treatment on the way to the emergency room.

If your symptoms go away after a few minutes, you may have had a TIA. Although brief, a TIA is a sign of a serious condition that will not go away without medical help.

Unfortunately, because TIAs clear up, many people ignore them. But paying attention to a TIA can save your life. Tell your health care team about your symptoms right away.

Treatment

Your stroke treatment begins the moment emergency medical services (EMS) arrives to take you to the hospital. Once at the hospital, you may receive emergency care, treatment to prevent another stroke, rehabilitation to treat the side effects of stroke, or all three.

On the way to the hospital

If someone you know shows signs of stroke, call 120 right away. The key to stroke treatment and recovery is getting to the hospital quickly. Yet 1 in 3 stroke patients never calls 120. Calling an ambulance means that medical staff can begin life-saving treatment on the way to the emergency room.

Stroke patients who are taken to the hospital in an ambulance may get diagnosed and treated more quickly than people who do not arrive in an ambulance. This is because emergency treatment starts on the way to the hospital. The emergency workers may take you to a specialized stroke center to ensure that you receive the quickest possible diagnosis and treatment. The emergency workers will also collect valuable information that guides treatment and alert hospital medical staff before you arrive at the emergency room, giving them time to prepare.

What happens at the hospital?

At the hospital, health professionals will ask about your medical history and about the time your symptoms started. Brain scans will show what type of stroke you had. You may also work with a neurologist who treats brain disorders, a neurosurgeon that performs surgery on the brain, or a specialist in another area of medicine.

If you get to the hospital within 3 hours of the first symptoms of an ischemic stroke, you may get a type of medicine called a thrombolytic (a "clot-busting" drug) to break up blood clots. Tissue plasminogen activator (tPA) is a thrombolytic. It improves the chances of recovering from a stroke. Studies show that patients with ischemic strokes who receive tPA are more likely to recover fully or have less disability than patients who do not receive the drug. Patients treated with tPA are also less likely to need long-term care in a nursing home. Unfortunately, many stroke victims don't get to the hospital in time for tPA treatment. This is why it's so important to recognize the signs and symptoms of stroke right away and call 120.

Medicine, surgery, or other procedures may be needed to stop the bleeding and save brain tissue. For example, endovascular procedures may be used to treat certain hemorrhagic strokes. The doctor inserts a long tube through a major artery in the leg or arm and then guides the tube to the site of the weak spot or break in a blood vessel. The tube is then used to install a device, such as a coil, to repair the damage or prevent bleeding. Hemorrhagic strokes may be treated with surgery. If the bleeding is caused by a ruptured aneurysm, a metal clip may be put in place to stop the blood loss.

What happens next?

If you have had a stroke, you are at high risk for another stroke. 1 of 4 stroke survivors has another stroke within 5 years. The risk of stroke within 90 days of a TIA may be as high as 17%, with the greatest risk during the first week.

That's why it's important to treat the underlying causes of stroke, including heart disease, high blood pressure, atrial fibrillation (fast, irregular heartbeat), high cholesterol, and diabetes. Your doctor may give you medications or tell you to change your diet, exercise, or adopt other healthy lifestyle habits. Surgery may also be helpful in some cases.

Recovering from stroke

Recovery time after a stroke is different for everyone—it can take weeks, months, or even years. Some people recover fully, but others have long-term or lifelong disabilities.

What to expect after a stroke?

If you have had a stroke, you can make great progress in regaining your independence. However, some problems may continue:

- paralysis (inability to move some parts of the body), weakness, or both on one side of the body

- trouble with thinking, awareness, attention, learning, judgment, and memory
- problems understanding or forming speech
- trouble controlling or expressing emotions
- numbness or strange sensations
- pain in the hands and feet that worsens with movement and temperature changes
- trouble with chewing and swallowing
- problems with bladder and bowel control
- depression

Stroke rehabilitation

Rehabilitation can include working with speech, physical, and occupational therapists. Speech therapy helps people who have problems producing or understanding speech. Physical therapy uses exercises to help you relearn movement and coordination skills you may have lost because of the stroke. Occupational therapy focuses on improving daily activities, such as eating, drinking, dressing, bathing, reading, and writing.

Therapy and medicine may help with depression or other mental health conditions following a stroke. Joining a patient support group may help you adjust to life after a stroke. Talk with your health care team about local support groups, or check with an area medical center. Support from family and friends can also help relieve fear and anxiety following a stroke. Let your loved ones know how you feel and what they can do to help you.

(1,627 words)

Task 1

Read the passage above and answer the following questions.

(1) What is stroke?

(2) What does stroke cause?

(3) What are different types of strokes?

(4) Which type of stroke is the most common one?

(5) What is an ischemic stroke?

(6) What is a hemorrhagic stroke?

(7) What conditions can cause hemorrhagic strokes?

(8) What is a transient ischemic attack?

(9) What are symptoms of stroke?

(10) What should you do if you think someone may be having a stroke?

(11) What is the key to stroke treatment and recovery?

(12) Why is it so important to recognize the signs and symptoms of stroke right away and call 120?

(13) How long does it take to recover from a stroke?

(14) What problems may continue after a stroke?

(15) What does stroke rehabilitation include?

Task 2

Read the following paragraph carefully and fill in the blanks with the words from the box.

swelling	leading	substance	flow	bleeding
cause	likely	risk	condition	pregnant

Stroke is not common in pregnancy or during the years women can have children. But pregnancy does put women at higher risk for stroke, and the rate of pregnancy-related stroke is rising. Sometimes problems that increase the (1)_____ for stroke can happen. First, having high blood pressure during pregnancy is the (2)_____ cause of stroke in pregnant women or women who have recently given birth. Some women who had healthy blood pressure levels before getting (3)_____ can develop high blood pressure during pregnancy. Second, preeclampsia(子痫前期) is a more severe type of high blood pressure during pregnancy. At its most severe, preeclampsia can (4)_____ seizures(子痫) and lead to stroke. Third, some women suddenly develop problems with blood sugar during pregnancy, a (5)_____ called gestational diabetes. Gestational diabetes raises the risk for high blood pressure during pregnancy and for heart disease and stroke later in life. Last, pregnancy makes the blood more (6)_____ to clot, which can lead to stroke. This increased risk for clotting happens in part because (7)_____ from pregnancy can reduce blood (8)_____ to the lower legs. During late pregnancy, the body also makes more of a (9)_____ that helps blood clot. This helps protect women from (10)_____ too much when they give birth, but it also raises the risk for stroke.

Task 3

Study the boldfaced words in each of the following sentences and make a sentence of your own.

(1) Blood clots often cause the blockages that **lead to** ischemic strokes.

Your sentence: The effects of acute blood loss are mainly due to the loss of intravascular volume, which can **lead to** cardiovascular collapse, shock, and death.

(2) Intracerebral hemorrhage **is the most common type of** hemorrhagic stroke.

Your sentence: _____

_____

(3) Recognizing and treating TIAs can **lower the risk of** a major stroke.

Your sentence: _____

_____

(4) Stroke patients may not **be eligible for** these if they don't arrive at the hospital in time.

Your sentence: _____

_____

(5) If the bleeding **is caused by** a ruptured aneurysm, a metal clip may be put in place to stop the blood loss.

Your sentence: _____

_____

(6) If you have had a stroke, you **are at a high risk for** another stroke.

Your sentence: _____

_____

Task 4

Reorder the following sentences into a reasonable paragraph.

(1) The experiment successfully implemented a brain-computer interface in monkeys, allowing them to control a robotic arm with their thoughts.

(2) China has successfully conducted the world's first brain-computer interface experiment on a non-human primate in Beijing, *Beijing Daily* reported.

(3) Brain-computer interface technology can help patients with conditions that cause motor dysfunction, such as stroke and ALS, improve their quality of life, said Ma Yongjie, a neurosurgeon at Beijing-based Xuanwu Hospital Capital Medical University.

(4) "The success of the first animal trial is a breakthrough from zero to one, but getting the success to the clinic is a process from 1 to 100, so we still have a long way to go," he said.

Correct order: ____　____　____　____

Story sharing

The following story① shares the author's personal experiences as a caregiver for her father, who was diagnosed with cerebral amyloid angiopathy before she graduated from medical school. She played a role both as a doctor and as a daughter in taking care of her father. Please read the story and then finish the tasks.

When I imagined this moment, I always thought that it would crush me. Dad stared at me and then back at the social worker. She stood in the doorway, smiling expectantly. She asked again, more loudly than necessary: "Can you introduce me, Paul?" She'd just started work at the nursing home, and I hadn't met her yet. Purple glasses swung from a chain around her neck. I took off my coat and put down my infant son's car seat. He snored quietly, shiny rivulets of drool wetting his chin.

"Yes, yes, this is ..." Dad trailed off. Sun filtered through the social worker's glasses, spilling light across Dad's face. He looked older than usual today, and his eyes seemed guarded in a way I hadn't noticed before. But they were the same pale blue eyes that would squint critically at my high school calculus homework at our old kitchen table. "Aha! I see you have an incorrect answer here," he'd say, and cross it out with a flourish. "Let's figure it out together." An engineer, he loved a good problem to chew on.

"This is, this is my sister Jean," he offered, blinking at me.

"No, no, Dad," I said quietly, taking his hand. "It's me, Audrey, your daughter." I sat on the edge of the bed. He smiled at me. Not in recognition—maybe in relief. I wasn't sure. I tried to blink away the tears rising in my eyes, waiting for him to reply, "Of course. This is Audrey, my daughter." But he never did.

Instead, my son broke the silence, red-faced and kicking. And with that, the moment I had dreaded for so long, the moment when my dad first did not recognize me, had passed. I pretended to smile and propped the baby up. Dad peered over at him and we remarked on his new teeth, so small and symmetrical and sharp. I sat in the car and cried before driving home.

My father's diagnosis came just before I graduated from medical school: cerebral amyloid angiopathy. Amyloid had weakened the blood vessels in his brain, leading to unrelenting hemorrhagic strokes. So I began a journey as a caregiver in two domains: as a doctor and as a daughter.

I started intern year as we all do. I'd stand at the foot of a bed and genuinely wonder: is

① Adapted from "Becoming a caregiver—lessons from my dad." Provenzano, A. M. (2018). *New England Journal of Medicine*, 379(18), 1696 – 1697.

this patient sick or not sick? I craved the pulsing crimson flash of a true arterial stick. I struggled each morning to present on rounds just right—not too much, forcing my resident to wheel her fingers in a circle, eyebrows arched, urging me to speed up; and not too little, leaving my attending with a flood of unanswered questions.

Not wishing to disturb me in the hospital with a phone call, Dad would summarize each episode of symptoms in succinct emails that he'd peck out with his index fingers, glasses sliding down his nose. After an attack in the grocery store, he wrote to me: "I reached into a freezer to get something. My hand ended up 6 inches below the target. With my left hand I pinched my upper arm, then my upper leg. Little sensitivity." He'd close each email admonishing me: "Do not be alarmed. I am fine." But I know the episodes scared him. A widower, he soon moved to Boston with his 70-lb Labrador Retriever to be closer to me and my brother.

By early senior year, I had learned some medicine. My dad telephoned and awoke me after call one afternoon, and when I went to see him, I could easily discern: he is sick. He is slumped in his chair, weak, face sagging. A few images from that night linger in my memory: the resident unfurling a blue drape over Dad's chest; the neurosurgeon's black Danskos, her right heel more worn than the left, as she paced outside Dad's room; the ED attending scrolling through Dad's head CT for me, grim and quiet. I saw the ugly white plume of blood, and I knew that everything would be different from then on.

Months passed. I accompanied Dad on an accelerating stream of hospitalizations, appointments, and rehab stays. Each time, I'd stand at his side and give a detailed history, his medication list in hand. But despite everything we did, I felt him slipping away. Usually so placid, he would become enraged when a Tupperware lid failed to seal under his trembling fingers and pasta salad rained down on the floor. The joy he found in walking his dog faded to fear as balance and strength drained from his legs. The bleeding soon left him unable to read. This seemed the ultimate cruelty, because he loved language. Before he got sick, as he read, he'd write down lists of obscure words to look up later. Even now when I pull one of his books from the shelf, often a bookmark covered in tidy rows of his angular, all-caps print will flutter to the floor.

And then the day came when Dad didn't know me. I felt lost.

At that point, there were few medical decisions to make. We had decided that there were to be no more appointments, no more hospitalizations, no more lab draws. I could no longer offer him my medical expertise. I wondered: what am I to him—if he doesn't know me as his daughter and my role in guiding his medical care is no longer necessary?

But our visits soon found a new rhythm. Sometimes he recognized me as his daughter and knew my name; sometimes he didn't. On his good days, he trusted me to brush his teeth and comb his hair. He'd close his eyes while the electric toothbrush whirred. He found it increasingly difficult to find any words to say, so I'd fill the silence by reading him news headlines from my phone. Sometimes I'd look up and see him watching me with a hint of his old smile. On days when he was sleepy, I'd play his most beloved CDs, hoping the familiar sighs of John Coltrane could somehow tether us together. My brother would come visit, and they'd binge-watch Dad's favorite TV shows, *Monk* and *Downton Abbey*. A massive frontal stroke, disrupting the brain's seat of restraint, holds few benefits, but for my dad, one became clear: he loved to eat, and his appetite knew no limit. On each visit I'd bring him an enormous dish of ice cream. "Chocolate!" he'd exclaim as I opened the bag. He would savor every bite, holding the cold, sweet cream on his tongue until it melted.

On what turned out to be his last birthday, Dad asked for a vanilla cake. My husband and I brought him outside. A cool September breeze rippled through the purple asters ringing the patio. Our son toddled around, picking up decorative white stones and placing them on the table. After singing and cake, Dad fell asleep in his wheelchair. When we took him back upstairs, I noticed that our son had slipped half a dozen of the little white stones onto his lap.

On his bad days, though, I'd hear Dad from the elevator, shouting down a menace conjured from his damaged brain. Sometimes the sight of my giggling son would calm him; most of the time, though, nothing could. I'd cower in the hallway, trying not to cry.

Then, Dad died, peacefully and comfortably. I didn't expect to feel anything, thinking I'd said goodbye to him years before, when he no longer knew me as his daughter. To my surprise, a harsh, raw anger erupted from somewhere within me. Each day I felt anew Dad's wrath at the pasta salad falling to the floor. Each weekend, when I'd typically go to see him, fury oozed from my pores.

(1,300 words)

Task 1

Read the passage above and write a paragraph to complete it, with the first sentence being provided.

It wasn't that I missed the visits, exactly.

_____

_____

_____

_____

_____

_____

_____

_____

_____

_____

_____

_____

_____

_____

_____

Task 2

Discuss the following questions in groups.

(1) Are hemorrhagic strokes unrelenting? Why or why not?

(2) What lessons can you learn from the author's role as a doctor?

(3) What lessons can you learn from the author's role as a daughter?

Vocabulary checklist

英文	中文
* lung [lʌŋ]	肺
* **cardiovascular** system [ˌkɑːdiəʊˈvæskjələ(r)]	心血管系统
* blood **vessel** [ˈvesl]	血管
* artery [ˈɑːtəri]	动脉
* vein [veɪn]	静脉
* hormone [ˈhɔːməʊn]	激素;荷尔蒙
* waste product	代谢废物

英文	中文
chamber [ˈtʃeɪmbə(r)]	(身体或器官的)室,腔
* ventricle [ˈventrɪkl]	心室
interventricular septum [ɪntəvenˈtrɪkjʊlə ˈseptəm]	室间隔
* atrium [ˈeɪtriəm]	心房
interatrial septum [ɪntərˈeɪtrɪəl]	房间隔
* atria [ˈeɪtriə]	心房(atrium 的复数)
atrioventricular valve [ˌeɪtrɪəʊvenˈtrɪkjʊlə(r)]	房室瓣
tricuspid valve [traɪˈkʌspɪd]	三尖瓣
mitral valve [ˈmaɪtrəl]	二尖瓣
pulmonic valve [pʌlˈmɒnɪk]	肺动脉瓣
* **pulmonary** artery [ˈpʌlmənəri]	肺动脉
aortic valve [eɪˈɔːtɪk]	主动脉瓣
* aorta [eɪˈɔːtə]	主动脉
* pulmonary circulation	肺循环
* **systemic** circulation [sɪˈstiːmɪk]	体循环
* pulmonary vein	肺静脉
oxygenated [ˈɒksɪdʒəneɪtɪd]	富含氧气的

英文	中文
* capillary [kəˈpɪləri]	毛细血管
superior **vena cava** [ˈviːnə ˈkeɪvə]	上腔静脉
inferior vena cava	下腔静脉
sinus (or **sinoatrial**) node [ˈsaɪnəs] [ˌsaɪnəuˈeɪtrɪəl]	窦房结
pacemaker	起搏点
atrioventricular (or AV) node	房室结
* systole [ˈsɪstəli]	收缩
* diastole [daɪˈæstəli]	舒张
spell	发作
* stroke [strəʊk]	脑卒中
* attack	突然发作
* ischemic [ɪsˈkɪmɪk]	缺血的
* hemorrhagic [ˌheməˈrædʒɪk]	出血的
* blood clot	血块
aneurysm [ˈænjərɪzəm]	动脉瘤
intracerebral hemorrhage [ˌɪntrəˈserəbrəl]	脑出血
subarachnoid hemorrhage [ˌsʌbəˈræknɔɪd]	蛛网膜下腔出血
* sign [saɪn]	体征
* symptom [ˈsɪmptəm]	症状

英文	中文
* numbness ['nʌmnəs]	麻木
* confusion [kən'fjuːʒn]	意识错乱
* dizziness ['dɪzɪnəs]	头晕
* coordination [kəʊˌɔːdɪ'neɪʃn]	协调
droop [druːp]	下垂
slurred [slɜːd]	发音含糊的
* rehabilitation [ˌriːəˌbɪlɪ'teɪʃn]	康复
* neurologist [njʊə'rɒlədʒɪst]	神经病学家
* neurosurgeon ['njʊərəʊsɜːdʒən]	神经外科医生
thrombolytic [ˌθrɒmbə'lɪtɪk]	血栓溶解剂
tissue **plasminogen** activator [plæz'mɪnədʒən]	组织型纤溶酶原激活物
nursing home	疗养院
endovascular procedure [ˌendəʊ'væskjʊlə]	血管内手术治疗
coil [kɔɪl]	(绳索、金属线等的)圈
metal clip	金属夹
atrial **fibrillation** [ˌfɪbrɪ'leɪʃən]	心房颤动
cholesterol [kə'lestərɒl]	胆固醇

英文	中文
* diabetes [ˌdaɪəˈbiːtiːz]	糖尿病
* bladder [ˈblædə(r)]	膀胱
occupational therapist	职业治疗师
* cerebral [səˈriːbrəl]	大脑的
amyloid [ˈæmɪlɔɪd]	淀粉样蛋白
angiopathy [ˌændʒɪˈɒpəθi]	血管病
* intern [ɪnˈtɜːn]	实习医师
arterial stick [ɑːˈtɪəriəl]	(采集)动脉血(标本)
* round	查房
* resident [ˈrezɪdənt]	住院医师
* attending [əˈtendɪŋ]	主治医师
* episode	发作
drape [dreɪp]	手术洞巾
* ED	急诊科(Emergency Department 的缩写)
lab draw	医疗化验
* frontal [ˈfrʌntl]	前额的

注：* 表示高频医学英语词汇。

Respiratory system

Upon completion of this chapter, you will be able to

❖ name the parts of the respiratory system and tell the functions of them;

❖ describe the process of respiration;

❖ list major pathologic conditions affecting the respiratory system;

❖ understand information about lung cancer;

❖ gather information about common diseases pertaining to the respiratory system;

❖ present one common respiratory disease with group members.

Theme reading 1

An introduction to the respiratory system[①]

What does the respiratory system do?

The respiratory system allows us to breathe. It brings oxygen into our bodies (called inspiration, or inhalation) and sends carbon dioxide out (called expiration, or exhalation). This exchange of oxygen and carbon dioxide is called respiration.

What are the parts of the respiratory system?

The respiratory system includes the nose, mouth, throat, voice box, windpipe, and lungs.

Air enters the respiratory system through the nose or the mouth. If it goes in the nostrils (also called nares), the air is warmed and humidified. Tiny hairs called cilia protect the nasal passageways and other parts of the respiratory tract, filtering out dust and other particles that enter the nose through the breathed air.

---

① Adapted from "Lung and Respiratory system." Hirsch, L. (2018). https://kidshealth.org

The two openings of the airway (the nasal cavity and the mouth) meet at the pharynx, or throat, at the back of the nose and mouth. The pharynx is part of the digestive system as well as the respiratory system because it carries both food and air.

At the bottom of the pharynx, this pathway divides into two, one for food—the esophagus, which leads to the stomach—and the other for air. The epiglottis, a small flap of tissue, covers the air-only passage when we swallow, keeping food and liquid from going into the lungs.

The larynx, or voice box, is the top part of the air-only pipe. This short tube contains a pair of vocal cords, which vibrate to make sounds.

The trachea, or windpipe, is the continuation of the airway below the larynx. The walls of the trachea are strengthened by stiff rings of cartilage to keep it open. The trachea is also lined with cilia, which sweep fluids and foreign particles out of the airway so that they stay out of the lungs.

At its bottom end, the trachea divides into left and right air tubes called bronchi, which connect to the lungs. Within the lungs, the bronchi branch into smaller bronchi and even smaller tubes called bronchioles. Bronchioles end in tiny air sacs called alveoli, where the exchange of oxygen and carbon dioxide actually takes place. Each person has hundreds of millions of alveoli in their lungs. This network of alveoli, bronchioles, and bronchi is known as the bronchial tree.

The lungs also contain elastic tissues that allow them to inflate and deflate without losing shape. They're covered by a thin lining called the pleura.

The chest cavity, or thorax, is the airtight box that houses the bronchial tree, lungs, heart, and other structures. The top and sides of the thorax are formed by the ribs and attached muscles, and the bottom is formed by a large muscle called the diaphragm. The chest walls form a protective cage around the lungs and other contents of the chest cavity.

How does the respiratory system work?

The cells in our bodies need oxygen to stay alive. Carbon dioxide is made in our bodies as cells do their jobs.

The respiratory system allow oxygen in the air to be taken into the body, while also letting the body get rid of carbon dioxide in the air breathed out.

When you breathe in, the diaphragm moves downward toward the abdomen, and the rib muscles pull the ribs upward and outward. This makes the chest cavity bigger and pulls air through the nose or mouth into the lungs.

In exhalation, the diaphragm moves upward and the chest wall muscles relax, causing the chest cavity to get smaller and push air out of respiratory system through the nose or mouth.

Every few seconds, with each inhalation, air fills a large portion of the millions of alveoli. In a process called diffusion, oxygen moves from the alveoli to the blood through the capillaries (tiny blood vessels) lining the alveolar walls. Once in the bloodstream, oxygen gets picked up by the hemoglobin in red blood cells. This oxygen-rich blood then flows back to the heart, which pumps it through the arteries to oxygen-hungry tissues throughout the body.

In the tiny capillaries of the body tissues, oxygen is freed from the hemoglobin and moves into the cells. Carbon dioxide, made by the cells as they do their work, moves out of the cells into the capillaries, where most of it dissolves in the plasma of the blood. Blood rich in carbon dioxide then returns to the heart via the veins. From the heart, this blood is pumped to the lungs, where carbon dioxide passes into the alveoli to be exhaled.

Tips to keep your lungs healthy

Sometimes we take our lungs for granted. They keep us alive and well and for the most part, we don't need to think about them. That's why it is important to prioritize your lung health.

Your body has a natural defense system designed to protect the lungs, keeping dirt and germs at bay. But there are some important things you can do to reduce your risk of lung disease. Here are some ways to keep your lungs healthy.

Don't smoke. Cigarette smoking is the major cause of lung cancer and chronic obstructive pulmonary disease. Cigarette smoke can narrow the air passages and make breathing more difficult. It causes chronic inflammation, or swelling in the lung, which can lead to chronic bronchitis. Over time cigarette smoke destroys lung tissue and may trigger changes that grow into cancer. If you smoke, it's never too late to benefit from quitting.

Avoid exposure to indoor pollutants that can damage your lungs. Secondhand smoke, chemicals in the home and workplace, and radon all can cause or worsen lung disease.

Minimize exposure to outdoor air pollution. The air quality outside can vary from day to day and sometimes is unhealthy to breathe. Knowing how outdoor air pollution affects your health and useful strategies to minimize prolonged exposure can help keep you and your family well.

Prevent infection. A cold or other respiratory infection can sometimes become very serious. There are several things you can do to protect yourself: Wash your hands often with soap and water; alcohol-based cleaners are a good substitute if you cannot wash. Avoid crowds during the cold and flu season. When a flu vaccine is available to you, we encourage you to utilize this safe and effective tool to prevent severe illness from occurring.

Get regular check-ups. Regular check-ups help prevent diseases, even when you are feeling well. This is especially true for lung disease, which sometimes goes undetected until it is serious.

Exercise regularly. Whether you are young or old, slender or large, able-bodied or living with a chronic illness or disability, being physically active can help keep your lungs healthy.

(1,108 words)

Task 1

Read the passage above and answer the following questions.

(1) What does the respiratory system do?

(2) What are the parts of the respiratory system?

(3) How do the diaphragm and rib muscles move during inhalation and exhalation?

(4) How does oxygen move from the lungs to the bloodstream?

(5) How can we keep our lungs healthy?

Task 2

Please label Figure 2-1 with the medical terms you've learnt in Theme reading 1.

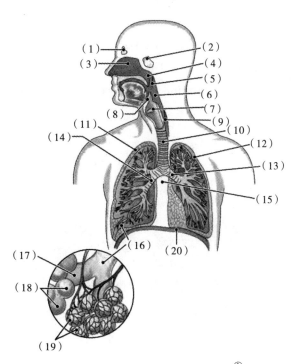

Figure 2-1   The respiratory system[1]

(1) frontal sinus	(2) sphenoidal sinus
(3)	(4)
(5)	(6)

---

[1] Adapted from *Medical terminology: an illustrated guide* (*7th edition*). Cohen, B. J., & DePetris, A. (2014). Philadelphia: Lippincott Williams & Wilkins.

(7)	(8)
(9)	(10)
(11)	(12)
(13)	(14)
(15) mediastinum	(16) terminal bronchiole
(17) alveolar duct	(18)
(19)	(20)

Task 3

The respiratory system works closely with the cardiovascular system to help our bodies absorb oxygen and eliminate carbon dioxide. The exchange of oxygen and carbon dioxide is called respiration (Figure 2-2). Please draw a mind map of respiration with the words and phrases in Theme reading 1 and Figure 2-2.

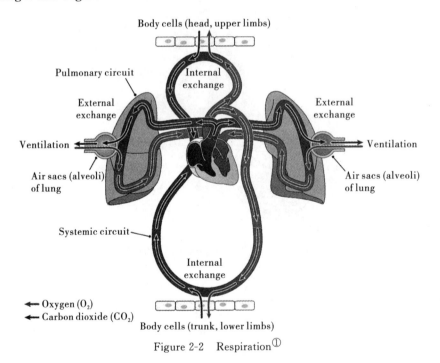

Figure 2-2　Respiration[1]

---

[1] Adapted from *Medical terminology: an illustrated guide* (*7th edition*). Cohen, B. J., & DePetris, A. (2014). Philadelphia: Lippincott Williams & Wilkins.

Vocabulary bridge

Study the following terms for common signs, symptoms and diseases related to the respiratory system and translate them into Chinese.

Medical terms	Explanation	Chinese translations
acidosis	excessive acidity of blood due to an accumulation of acids or an excessive loss of bicarbonate	酸中毒
anoxia	total absence of oxygen in body tissues	
atelectasis	collapse of lung tissue, preventing respiratory exchange of oxygen (O_2) and carbon dioxide (CO_2)	
empyema	pus in a body cavity, especially in the pleural cavity (pyothorax)	
epistaxis	hemorrhage from the nose; also called nosebleed	
hypoxemia	deficiency of oxygen in the blood, usually a sign of respiratory impairment	
hypoxia	deficiency of oxygen in body tissues, usually a sign of respiratory impairment	
influenza	acute, contagious respiratory infection characterized by sudden onset of fever, chills, headache, and muscle pain	
lung cancer	pulmonary malignancy commonly attributable to cigarette smoking	
pertussis	acute infectious disease characterized by a "whoop"-sounding cough; also called whooping cough	
pleural effusion	abnormal presence of fluid in the pleural cavity	
pneumothorax	collection of air in the pleural cavity, causing the complete or partial collapse of a lung	

Theme reading 2

Lung cancer[1]

What is lung cancer?

Cancer is a disease in which cells in the body grow out of control. When cancer starts in the lungs, it is called lung cancer.

Lung cancer begins in the lungs and may spread to lymph nodes or other organs in the body, such as the brain. Cancer from other organs also may spread to the lungs. When cancer

---

[1] Adapted from "About lung cancer" (n. d.). https://www.cdc.gov

cells spread from one organ to another, they are called metastases.

Types of lung cancer

The two main types of lung cancer are small cell lung cancer (SCLC) and non-small cell lung cancer (NSCLC). These categories refer to what the cancer cells look like under a microscope. Non-small cell lung cancer is more common than small cell lung cancer. The most common sub-types of NSCLC based on histology are adenocarcinoma, squamous cell carcinoma and large cell carcinoma.

The histology of lung cancer can be determined by a pathologist who looks at a sample of your tumor with a microscope.

The risk factors for lung cancer

Smoking

Cigarette smoking is the number one risk factor for lung cancer. In the United States, cigarette smoking is linked to about 80% to 90% of lung cancer deaths. Using other tobacco products such as cigars or pipes also increases the risk for lung cancer. Tobacco smoke is a toxic mix of more than 7,000 chemicals. Many are poisons. At least 70 are known to cause cancer in people or animals.

People who smoke cigarettes are 15 to 30 times more likely to get lung cancer or die from lung cancer than people who do not smoke. Even smoking a few cigarettes a day or smoking occasionally increases the risk of lung cancer. The more years a person smokes and the more cigarettes smoked each day, the more risk goes up.

People who quit smoking have a lower risk of lung cancer than if they had continued to smoke, but their risk is higher than the risk for people who never smoked. Quitting smoking at any age can lower the risk of lung cancer.

Cigarette smoking can cause cancer almost anywhere in the body. Cigarette smoking causes cancer of the mouth and throat, esophagus, stomach, colon, rectum, liver, pancreas, voice box (larynx), trachea, bronchus, kidney and renal pelvis, urinary bladder, and cervix, and causes acute myeloid leukemia.

Secondhand smoke

Smoke from other people's cigarettes, pipes, or cigars (secondhand smoke) also causes lung cancer. When a person breathes in secondhand smoke, it is like he or she is smoking. In the United States, one out of four people who don't smoke, including 14 million children, were exposed to secondhand smoke during 2013 – 2014.

Radon

Radon is a naturally occurring gas that comes from rocks and dirt and can get trapped in houses and buildings. It cannot be seen, tasted, or smelled. According to the U. S. Environmental Protection Agency (EPA), external icon radon causes about 21,000 cases of lung cancer each year, making it the second leading cause of lung cancer. Nearly one out of every 15 homes in the United States is thought to have high radon levels. The EPA recommends testing homes for radon and using proven ways to lower high radon levels.

Other substances

Examples of substances found at some workplaces that increase risk include asbestos, arsenic, diesel exhaust, and some forms of silica and chromium. For many of these substances, the risk of getting lung cancer is even higher for those who smoke.

Personal or family history of lung cancer

If you are a lung cancer survivor, there is a risk that you may develop another lung cancer, especially if you smoke. Your risk of lung cancer may be higher if your parents, brothers or sisters, or children have had lung cancer. This could be true because they also smoke, or they live or work in the same place where they are exposed to radon and other substances that can cause lung cancer.

The symptoms of lung cancer

Different people have different symptoms for lung cancer. Some people have symptoms related to the lungs. Some people whose lung cancer has spread to other parts of the body (metastasized) have symptoms specific to that part of the body. Some people just have general symptoms of not feeling well. It is true that most people with lung cancer don't have symptoms until the cancer is advanced. Lung cancer symptoms may include

- coughing that gets worse or doesn't go away;
- chest pain;
- shortness of breath;
- wheezing;
- coughing up blood;
- feeling very tired all the time;
- weight loss with no known cause.

Other changes that can sometimes occur with lung cancer may include repeated bouts of pneumonia and swollen or enlarged lymph nodes (glands) inside the chest in the area between the lungs.

Symptoms of lung cancer are the same for smokers and nonsmokers. Some people have general symptoms of not feeling well or feeling tired all the time. Some people cough frequently, cough up blood, or have chest pain, wheezing, or shortness of breath.

These symptoms can happen with other illnesses. If you have any of these symptoms, talk to your doctor, who can help find the cause.

Screening for lung cancer

Screening means testing for a disease when there are no symptoms or history of that disease. Doctors recommend a screening test to find a disease early, when treatment may work better.

The only recommended screening test for lung cancer is low-dose computed tomography (also called a low-dose CT scan, or LDCT). During an LDCT scan, you lie on a table and an

X-ray machine uses a low dose (amount) of radiation to make detailed images of your lungs. The scan only takes a few minutes and is not painful.

Who should be screened?

The U. S. Preventive Services Task Force (USPSTF) recommends external icon yearly lung cancer screening with LDCT for people who have a 20 pack-year or more smoking history, and smoke now or have quit within the past 15 years, and are between 50 and 80 years old.

A pack-year is smoking an average of one pack of cigarettes per day for one year. For example, a person could have a 20 pack-year history by smoking one pack a day for 20 years or two packs a day for 10 years.

Lung cancer screening has risks. Radiation from repeated LDCT tests can cause cancer in otherwise healthy people.

Staging of lung cancer

After lung cancer is diagnosed, doctors will determine the type of lung cancer patients have and the stage of the disease. Staging is based on the tumor's size, location, and evidence of spread to lymph nodes and other organs. Staging is needed to help determine your treatment plan.

Non-small cell lung cancer

The staging system most often used for NSCLC is the American Joint Committee on Cancer (AJCC) TNM system, which is based on 3 key pieces of information:

• The size and extent of the main tumor (T): How large is the tumor? Has it grown into nearby structures or organs?

• The spread to nearby lymph nodes (N): Has the cancer spread to nearby lymph nodes?

• The spread (metastasis) to distant sites (M): Has the cancer spread to distant organs such as the brain, bones, adrenal glands, liver, or the other lung?

The earliest stage of NSCLC is stage 0 (also called carcinoma in situ, or CIS). Other stages range from I (1) through IV (4). As a rule, the lower the number, the less the cancer has spread. A higher number, such as stage IV, means cancer has spread more. And within a stage, an earlier letter (or number) means a lower stage. Although each person's cancer experience is unique, cancers with similar stages tend to have a similar outlook and are often treated in much the same way.

Small-cell lung cancer

The stage of SCLC is based on the results of physical exams, biopsies, imaging tests, and any other tests that have been done for lung cancer. For treatment purposes, most doctors use a 2-stage system that divides SCLC into limited stage and extensive stage.

Limited-stage SCLC is cancer present in only one lung, which may have spread to surrounding lymph nodes. Treatment for limited-stage SCLC generally involves both chemotherapy and radiation therapy.

Extensive-stage SCLC is cancer that has spread to both lungs, lymph nodes far from the original cancer, or other parts of the body. As with other advanced cancers, extensive-stage SCLC is generally not curable, but there are treatments available that may help you live better and longer.

Treatment

Lung cancer is treated in several ways, depending on the type of lung cancer and how far it has spread. People with non-small cell lung cancer can be treated with surgery, chemotherapy, radiation therapy, targeted therapy, or a combination of these treatments. People with small cell lung cancer are usually treated with radiation therapy and chemotherapy.

• Surgery: An operation where doctors cut out cancer tissue.

• Chemotherapy: Using special medicines to shrink or kill the cancer cells. The drugs can be pills you take or medicines given in your veins, or sometimes both.

• Radiation therapy: Using high-energy rays (similar to X-rays) to kill the cancer cells.

• Targeted therapy: Using drugs to block the growth and spread of cancer cells. The drugs can be pills you take or medicines given in your veins.

Complementary and alternative medicine are medicines and health practices that are not standard cancer treatments. Complementary medicine is used in addition to standard treatments. Examples include acupuncture, dietary supplements, massage therapy, hypnosis, and meditation. Alternative medicine is used instead of standard treatments. Examples include special diets, megadose vitamins, herbal preparations, special teas, and magnet therapy.

Doctors from different specialties often work together to treat lung cancer. Pulmonologists are doctors who are experts in diseases of the lungs. Surgeons are doctors who perform operations. Thoracic surgeons specialize in chest, heart, and lung surgery. Medical oncologists are doctors who treat cancer with medicines. Radiation oncologists are doctors who treat cancers with radiation.

(1,660 words)

Task 1

Read the passage above and answer the following questions.

(1) What is lung cancer?

(2) What are types of lung cancer?

(3) What are the risk factors for lung cancer?

(4) Why is there lung cancer among people who never smoked?

(5) What are the symptoms of lung cancer?

(6) What are the symptoms of lung cancer among people who never smoked?

(7) Who should be screened?

(8) How are the stages of lung cancer determined?

(9) What are the stages of lung cancer?

(10) What are the treatments of lung cancer?

Task 2

Read the following paragraph carefully and fill in the blanks with the words from the box.

exhausted	uncommon	involve	prior	accessible
effectiveness	informed	concerned	particular	conducted

When people are diagnosed with lung cancer, doctors may discuss with patients whether or not a clinical trial is a good treatment option for them. Clinical trials are medical research studies that test the safety and (1)_____ of promising approaches to disease prevention, diagnosis, treatment and care. Clinical trials that test cancer treatments might (2)_____ the use of drugs, radiation therapy, surgery or other treatment methods. Treatments are only brought to clinical trials after significant (3)_____ research shows they have promise. These trials are carefully (4)_____ by doctors and trained teams to ensure that patients receive the best possible treatment and care. Some people think they should consider a clinical trial only after they've (5)_____ standard lung cancer treatment options. However, no matter where you are in your treatment process, there may be a clinical trial that is right for you. In fact, many trials are (6)_____ for people who have just been diagnosed or who have early-stage lung cancer. People are also sometimes (7)_____ that if they participate in a clinical trial they might only get a "sugar pill" (placebo) and not get any treatment at all. In fact, all patients participating in cancer clinical trials receive the best cancer treatment currently known for their type and stage of cancer. If placebos are used, patients usually receive them in addition to standard, proven treatments. Placebos may also be used when testing a new treatment for a (8)_____ type or stage of disease for which no standard treatments are available, but this is (9)_____ in cancer clinical trials. If a placebo will be used in a trial, patients are fully (10)_____ .

Task 3

Study the boldfaced words in each of the following sentences and make a sentence of your own.

(1) In the United States, one out of four people who don't smoke, including 14 million children, **were exposed to** secondhand smoke during 2013 – 2014.

Your sentence: <u>People who **are exposed to** radon and other substances also have a high risk of developing lung cancer.</u>

(2) These categories **refer to** what the cancer cells look like under a microscope.

Your sentence: _____

_____

(3) A tumor up to 5 cm wide that has not spread to any lymph nodes or other organs **is classified as** stage I.

Your sentence: _____

_____

(4) Lung cancer is treated in several ways, **depending on** how far it has spread.

Your sentence: _____

_____

(5) Thoracic surgeons **specialize in** chest, heart, and lung surgery.

Your sentence: _____

_____

(6) Researchers estimate that secondhand smoke **contributes to** about 7,300 and radon external icon to about 2,900 of these lung cancers.

Your sentence: _____

_____

Task 4

Reorder the following sentences into a reasonable paragraph.

(1) Their research played an important role in the global fight against respiratory disease, including severe acute respiratory syndrome (SARS), chronic obstructive pulmonary disease, lung cancer, etc.

(2) With nearly five decades of respiratory research and clinical experience between them, Zhong and two other team leaders, He Jianxin and Ran Pixi, led the group in working on many difficult respiratory ailments.

(3) The research team headed by Zhong Nanshan, one of the country's leading pulmonologists, received the 2020 State Scientific and Technological Progress Award's Innovation Team Award.

(4) Testament to its effectiveness is that doctors have been able to increase survival rates to over 90 percent for lung cancer patients five years after they have the surgery.

(5) The team's philosophy of "early detection, diagnosis, examination and treatment" has been widely adopted in China.

Correct order: ____ ____ ____ ____ ____

Story sharing

The following story[①] is written by Jennifer, a lung cancer survivor who shares her diagnosis, treatment, family and community support, and mindset. She also gives advice to other people living with lung cancer. Please read the story and finish the tasks.

A year and a half ago, I was feeling terribly run down and getting very winded from normal activities in spite of being fit and athletic. I was coughing, having trouble catching my breath, and experiencing some mild wheezing. These symptoms led me to my primary care physician, and when I didn't feel better on antibiotics within a few days, she ordered a chest X-ray.

On a busy Saturday, I let my husband Andy manage our kids' sports schedules and walked myself into the emergency department, expecting a case of walking pneumonia or bronchitis. Nothing could have surprised me more that day than to learn that I have Stage IV metastatic lung cancer.

As a lifelong athlete through college and now just "for fun," I couldn't understand how someone who follows a healthy diet, exercises regularly, and competes in triathlon and running events could possibly have incurable lung cancer.

I fought during the next month to become well enough to begin chemotherapy, knowing that statistically I would be an outlier if I could survive beyond a year or two. But 17 months after diagnosis, I am living very well as I continue chemo to keep the cancer in my lungs stable. The cancer that was found initially in my adrenal gland and liver is now undetectable.

Unfortunately, debilitating headaches and vomiting six months ago led to the identification of two lesions in my brain. Both were successfully removed via craniotomy. Four months later, as I was once again feeling my "new normal," MRI identified another brain lesion, which was successfully treated with stereotactic radiosurgery. I have recovered from these detours and use them as an opportunity to refocus on my overall wellness—which I know not to take for granted. I have maintenance chemotherapy every three weeks and MRI of

---

① Adapted from https://www.lungcancerresearchfoundation.org/jennifer/

my brain every few months to check for cancer growth. Despite these challenges, I have been determined to take control of the only thing that I can control: my mindset and gratitude each day.

Today, I have resumed most of my normal activities while working around many side effects and appointments: managing the household and parenting our 15-, 12-; and 10-year-old; coaching (and playing) volleyball; practicing yoga and walking our dogs; volunteering at my children's school and enjoying the daily joys of carpools and family dinners.

I am constantly challenged to accept the limitations that living with lung cancer places on my life and the emotional fear that can easily take hold if I am not vigilant in choosing to focus on the beauty in each day rather than worrying about the days to come. I work very hard to draw from my faith, practicing meditation focusing on how great my life is rather than how terrible my diagnosis is.

I have become as knowledgeable as possible about lung cancer in order to advocate for myself with all the members of my medical team, and I eagerly pay attention to research findings that I hope will help me and many others live better and longer with lung cancer.

Andy, my amazing husband of 22 years, has been instrumental in helping us navigate life with lung cancer, as have our parents and siblings. My sister (a nurse) and countless members of our community have supported me in so many ways: meals, play dates for the kids, a volleyball tournament fundraiser, encouraging emails/text messages/phone calls, and joining me to walk the 2016 Kansas City Free to Breathe 5K and helping our Team Gratitude raise the second greatest amount of money of any team at the event this year.

I feel an urgency to share information about lung cancer since it is so largely overlooked, especially in light of the fact that lung cancer claims more lives each year than breast, colon and prostate cancer combined. I tell my story to anyone who will listen, hoping that I can be part of a movement to increase funding for lung cancer research so that it might one day receive funding proportionate to the impact it has when compared with other cancers.

Lung cancer does not discriminate; financial support shouldn't either.

No one deserves lung cancer, and I want to help end the negative stigma unfairly attached to lung cancer and help raise funding to find a cure. I hope to increase my advocacy efforts now that I am back on a predictable schedule of chemo every three weeks. I know that for me and many others, we are in a race between our cancer growth and research breakthroughs.

In the short time since my diagnosis in April 2015, the landscape has changed tremendously as researchers discover new breakthroughs. The options are broader for anyone diagnosed today. I encourage anyone living with lung cancer to ask questions of doctors or reputable organizations; to access palliative care, psychology, nutrition and other resources to complement oncology; to ignore the larger Internet or "hearsay" information; and to focus on how you can make each day beautiful.

(829 words)

Task 1

Read the above passage and write a paragraph to complete it, with the first sentence provided.

Living with cancer forces patients to acknowledge how little control we each have, but the one thing we can control is the attitude we carry and share with others.

_____

_____

_____

_____

_____

_____

_____

_____

_____

Task 2

Discuss the following questions in groups.

(1) What did the author go through after she was diagnosed with lung cancer?

(2) Why did she find it urgent for her to share information about lung cancer?

(3) What advice did she give to the people with lung cancer?

(4) What lessons can you learn from the author's mindset after the diagnosis?

Vocabulary checklist

英文	中文
* **respiratory** system [rəˈspɪrətri]	呼吸系统
inspiration [ˌɪnspəˈreɪʃn]	吸气
* inhalation [ˌɪnhəˈleɪʃn]	吸入

英文	中文
expiration [ˌekspəˈreɪʃn]	呼气
＊ exhalation [ˌekshəˈleɪʃn]	呼出
＊ respiration [ˌrespəˈreɪʃn]	呼吸
voice box	喉
＊ windpipe [ˈwɪndpaɪp]	气管
nostril [ˈnɒstrəl]	鼻孔
nares [ˈneəriːz]	鼻孔（naris 的复数）
cilia [ˈsɪliə]	纤毛
＊ pharynx [ˈfærɪŋks]	咽
＊ esophagus [iːˈsɒfəgəs]	食管，食道
＊ epiglottis [ˌepɪˈglɒtɪs]	会厌
＊ larynx [ˈlærɪŋks]	喉
vocal **cord** [kɔːd]	声带
＊ trachea [trəˈkiːə]	气管
＊ cartilage [ˈkɑːtɪlɪdʒ]	软骨
＊ bronchi [ˈbrɒŋkaɪ]	支气管（bronchus 的复数）
＊ bronchiole [ˈbrɒŋkiəʊl]	细支气管

英文	中文
* air **sac** [sæk]	肺泡
* alveoli [æl'vi:əlaɪ]	肺泡（alveolus 的复数）
bronchial tree ['brɒŋkiəl]	支气管树
inflate [ɪn'fleɪt]	使充气
deflate [ˌdiː'fleɪt]	放气
* pleura ['plʊərə]	胸膜
* thorax ['θɔːræks]	胸，胸廓
* diaphragm ['daɪəfræm]	横膈
* abdomen ['æbdəmən]	腹，腹部
diffusion [dɪ'fjuːʒn]	扩散
* capillary [kə'pɪləri]	毛细血管
* hemoglobin [ˌhiːmə'gləʊbɪn]	血红蛋白
dissolve [dɪ'zɒlv]	溶解，分解
* plasma ['plæzmə]	血浆
* exhale [eks'heɪl]	呼出
chronic **obstructive pulmonary** disease (COPD) [əb'strʌktɪv] ['pʌlmənəri]	慢性阻塞性肺疾病
* bronchitis [brɒŋ'kaɪtɪs]	支气管炎

英文	中文
radon [ˈreɪdɒn]	氡
lymph node [lɪmf]	淋巴结
* metastases [məˈtæstəsiːz]	转移(metastasis 的复数)
* histology [hɪˈstɒlədʒi]	组织学
adenocarcinoma [ˌædɪnəʊˌkɑːsɪˈnəʊmə]	腺癌
squamous cell carcinoma [ˈskweɪməs]	鳞状细胞癌
* pathologist [pəˈθɒlədʒɪst]	病理学家,病理医生
* colon [ˈkəʊlən]	结肠
* rectum [ˈrektəm]	直肠
* pancreas [ˈpæŋkriəs]	胰腺
renal pelvis [ˈriːnl ˈpelvɪs]	肾盂
* urinary bladder [ˈjʊərɪnəri ˈblædə(r)]	膀胱
* cervix [ˈsɜːvɪks]	子宫颈
* acute **myeloid leukemia** [ˈmaɪəlɔɪd] [luːˈkɪːmɪə]	急性髓细胞性白血病
asbestos [æsˈbestɒs]	石棉
arsenic [ˈɑːsnɪk]	砷
diesel exhaust [ˈdiːzl ɪgˈzɔːst]	柴油机废气,柴油机尾气

英文	中文
silica [ˈsɪlɪkə]	二氧化硅
chromium [ˈkrəʊmiəm]	铬
wheezing [wiːzɪŋ]	气喘
bout [baʊt]	发作
* pneumonia [njuːˈməʊniə]	肺炎
* gland [ɡlænd]	腺
* low-dose computed **tomography**（LDCT） [təˈmɒɡrəfi]	低剂量计算机断层扫描
* **adrenal** gland [əˈdriːnl]	肾上腺
carcinoma in situ [ˌkɑːsɪˈnəʊmə]	原位癌
* biopsy [ˈbaɪɒpsi]	活组织检查
imaging test	影像检查
* chemotherapy [ˌkiːməʊˈθerəpi]	化疗
* **radiation** therapy [ˌreɪdiˈeɪʃn]	放射治疗
targeted therapy	靶向疗法
* acupuncture [ˈækjupʌŋktʃə(r)]	针灸
dietary supplement	膳食补充剂
* massage [ˈmæsɑːʒ]	按摩

英文	中文
hypnosis [hɪpˈnəʊsɪs]	催眠,催眠术
megadose [ˈmegəˌdəʊz]	高剂量
herbal preparation	中草药制剂
magnet therapy [ˈmæɡnət]	磁疗
pulmonologist [ˌpʌlməˈnɒlədʒɪst]	胸腔内科医生,肺病学家
thoracic surgeon [θɔːˈræsɪk]	胸腔外科医生
oncologist [ɒŋˈkɒlədʒɪst]	肿瘤学家,肿瘤医师
metastatic [ˌmetəˈstætɪk]	转移性的
* vomiting [ˈvɒmɪtɪŋ]	呕吐
* lesion [ˈliːʒn]	损害,病变
craniotomy [ˌkreɪnɪˈɒtəmi]	颅骨切开术
stereotactic radiosurgery [ˌstɪərɪəʊˈtæktɪk]	立体定向放射外科
prostate cancer [ˈprɒsteɪt]	前列腺癌
palliative care [ˈpæliətɪv]	姑息治疗
oncology [ɒŋˈkɒlədʒi]	肿瘤学

注：＊表示高频医学英语词汇。

Digestive system

Upon completion of this chapter, you will be able to

❖ name the organs of the digestive system, and describe the function of each;

❖ describe digestive process;

❖ list major pathologic conditions affecting the digestive system;

❖ understand information about liver cancer;

❖ gather information about common diseases in digestive system;

❖ present one common disease in digestive system with group members.

Theme reading 1

An introduction to the digestive system[①]

What is the digestive system?

Food is our fuel, and its nutrients give our bodies' cells the energy and substances they need to work. But before food can do that, it must be digested into small pieces the body can absorb and use.

The first step in the digestive process happens before we even taste food. Just by smelling that homemade apple pie or thinking about how delicious that ripe tomato is going to be, you start salivating—and the digestive process begins in preparation for that first bite.

Almost all animals have a tube-type digestive system in which food enters the mouth, passes through a long tube, and exits the body as feces (poop) through the anus.

Along the way, food is broken down into tiny molecules so that the body can absorb nutrients it needs:

---

① Adapted from "Digestive system." Hirsch, L. (2018). https://kidshealth.org

- Protein must be broken down into amino acids.
- Starches break down into simple sugars.
- Fats break down into fatty acids and glycerol.

The waste parts of food that the body can't use are what leave the body as feces.

How does digestion work?

The digestive system is made up of the alimentary canal (also called the digestive tract) and other organs, such as the liver and pancreas. The alimentary canal is the long tube of organs—including the esophagus, stomach, and intestines—that runs from the mouth to the anus. An adult's digestive tract is about 30 feet (about 9 meters) long.

Digestion begins in the mouth, well before food reaches the stomach. When we see, smell, taste, or even imagine a tasty meal, our salivary glands in front of the ear, under the tongue, and near the lower jaw begin making saliva (spit).

As the teeth tear and chop the food, spit moistens it for easy swallowing. A digestive enzyme in saliva called amylase starts to break down some of the carbohydrates (starches and sugars) in the food even before it leaves the mouth.

Swallowing, done by muscle movements in the tongue and mouth, moves the food into the throat, or pharynx. The pharynx is a passageway for food and air. A soft flap of tissue called the epiglottis closes over the windpipe when we swallow to prevent choking.

From the throat, food travels down a muscular tube in the chest called the esophagus. Waves of muscle contractions called peristalsis force food down through the esophagus to the stomach. A person normally isn't aware of the movements of the esophagus, stomach, and intestine that take place as food passes through the digestive tract.

At the end of the esophagus, a muscular ring or valve called a sphincter allows food to enter the stomach and then squeezes shut to keep food or fluid from flowing back up into the esophagus. The stomach muscles churn and mix the food with digestive juices that have acids and enzymes, breaking it into much smaller and digestible pieces. An acidic environment is needed for the digestion that takes place in the stomach.

By the time food is ready to leave the stomach, it has been processed into a thick liquid called chyme. A walnut-sized muscular valve at the outlet of the stomach called the pylorus keeps chyme in the stomach until it reaches the right consistency to pass into the small intestine. Chyme is then squirted down into the small intestine, where digestion of food continues so the body can absorb the nutrients into the bloodstream.

The small intestine is made up of three parts: the duodenum, the C-shaped first part; the jejunum, the coiled midsection; the ileum, the final section that leads into the large intestine.

The inner wall of the small intestine is covered with millions of microscopic, finger-like projections called villi. The villi are the vehicles through which nutrients can be absorbed into the blood. The blood then brings these nutrients to the rest of the body.

The liver (under the ribcage in the right upper part of the abdomen), the gall bladder (hidden just below the liver), and the pancreas (beneath the stomach) are not part of the alimentary canal, but these organs are essential to digestion.

The liver makes bile, which helps the body absorb fat. Bile is stored in the gall bladder until it is needed. The pancreas makes enzymes that help digest proteins, fats, and carbs. It also makes a substance that neutralizes stomach acid. These enzymes and bile travel through special pathways (called ducts) into the small intestine, where they help to break down food. The liver also helps process nutrients in the bloodstream.

From the small intestine, undigested food (and some water) travels to the large intestine through a muscular ring or valve that prevents food from returning to the small intestine. By the time food reaches the large intestine, the work of absorbing nutrients is nearly finished. The large intestine's main job is to remove water from the undigested matter and form solid waste (poop) to be excreted.

The large intestine has three parts. The cecum is the beginning of the large intestine. The appendix, a small, hollow, finger-like pouch, hangs at the end of the cecum. Scientists believe the appendix is left over from a previous time in human evolution.

The colon extends from the cecum up the right side of the abdomen, across the upper abdomen, and then down the left side of the abdomen, finally connecting to the rectum. The colon has three parts: the ascending colon, the transverse colon, which absorbs fluids and salts and the descending colon, which holds the resulting waste. The waste material passes into the S-shaped sigmoid colon and is stored in the rectum until eliminated through the anus.

The rectum is where feces are stored until they leave the digestive system through the anus as a bowel movement.

It takes hours for our bodies to fully digest food.

(965 words)

Task 1

Read the passage above and answer the following questions.

(1) What does the digestive system do?

(2) What is the digestive process that almost all animals have?

(3) What organs are involved in the digestive system?

(4) What are the parts of the small intestine?

(5) What are the parts of the large intestine?

Task 2

Please label Figure 3-1 with the medical terms you've learnt in Theme reading 1.

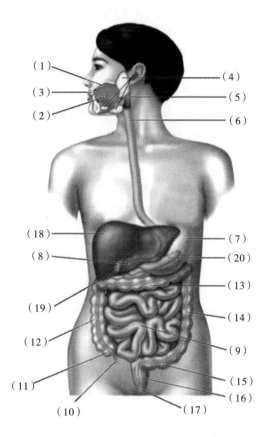

Figure 3-1　Digestive system[1]

(1)mouth	(2)tongue
(3)teeth	(4)
(5)	(6)
(7)	(8)
(9)	(10)
(11)	(12)
(13)	(14)
(15)	(16)

①Adapted from *Medical terminology: an illustrated guide (7th edition)*. Cohen, B. J., & DePetris, A. (2014). Philadelphia: Lippincott Williams & Wilkins.

(17)	(18)
(19)	(20)

Task 3

Figure 3-2 is a flow chart that traces the digestive process. Please describe the process in your own words using the arrows and the key words in the chart as the clues.

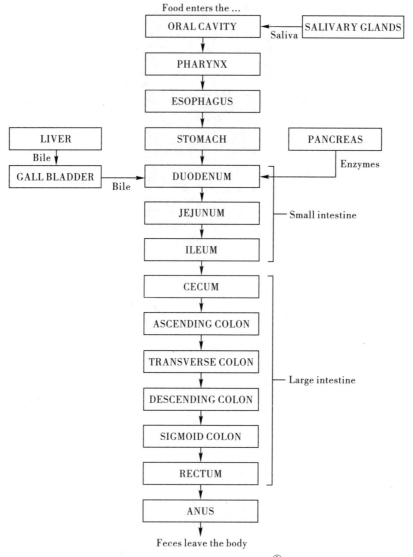

Figure 3-2　Digestive process[1]

---

[1] Adapted from *The language of medicine (10th edition)*. Chabner, D-E. (2014). Amsterdam: Saunders/Elsevier

_____

_____

_____

_____

_____

_____

_____

_____

_____

Vocabulary bridge

Study the following terms for common signs, symptoms and diseases related to the digestive system and translate them into Chinese.

Medical terms	Explanation	Chinese translations
appendicitis	inflammation of the appendix, which is usually acute and caused by blockage of the appendix followed by infection	阑尾炎
ascites	abnormal accumulation of serous fluid in the peritoneal cavity	
borborygmus	gurgling or rumbling sound heard over the large intestine that is caused by gas moving through the intestines	
cirrhosis	chronic liver disease characterized by destruction of liver cells that eventually leads to ineffective liver function and jaundice	
diverticular disease	condition in which bulging pouches (diverticula) in the gastrointestinal (GI) tract push the mucosal lining through the surrounding muscle	
dysentery	inflammation of the intestine, especially of the colon, which may be caused by chemical irritants, bacteria, protozoa, or parasites	
fistula	abnormal passage from one organ to another, or from a hollow organ to the surface	
gastroesophageal reflux disease (GERD)	backflow (reflux) of gastric contents into the esophagus due to malfunction of the lower esophageal sphincter (LES). Symptoms of GERD include heartburn (burning sensation caused by regurgitation of hydrochloric acid from the stomach to the esophagus), belching, and regurgitation of food	

Medical terms	Explanation	Chinese translations
hematochezia	passage of stools containing bright red blood	
hemorrhoid	mass of enlarged, twisted varicose veins in the mucous membrane inside (internal) or just outside (external) the rectum; also known as piles	
hernia	protrusion or projection of an organ or a part of an organ through the wall of the cavity that normally contains it	
inflammatory bowel disease (IBD)	ulceration of the colon mucosa. Chronic IBD of the colon is characterized by episodes of diarrhea, rectal bleeding, and pain	
Crohn disease	Crohn disease is distinguished from closely related bowel disorders by its inflammatory pattern, which tends to be patchy or segmented; also called regional colitis	
irritable bowel syndrome (IBS)	condition characterized by gastrointestinal signs and symptoms, including constipation, diarrhea, gas, and bloating, all in the absence of organic pathology; also called spastic colon	
jaundice	yellow discoloration of the skin, mucous membranes, and sclerae of the eyes caused by excessive levels of bilirubin in the blood (hyperbilirubinemia)	
obesity	condition in which a person accumulates an amount of fat that exceeds the body's skeletal and physical standards, usually an increase of 20 percent or more above ideal body weight	
polyp	small, tumorlike, benign growth that projects from a mucous membrane surface	
polyposis	condition in which polyps develop in the intestinal tract	
ulcer	open sore or lesion of the skin or mucous membrane accompanied by sloughing of inflamed necrotic tissue	
volvulus	twisting of the bowel on itself, causing obstruction	

Theme reading 2

Liver cancer[①]

What is liver cancer?

Primary liver cancer is a disease in which malignant (cancer) cells form in the tissues of the liver. Cancer that forms in other parts of the body and spreads to the liver is not primary

---

① Adapted from "Liver Cancer" (n. d.). https://medlineplus.gov

liver cancer. The liver is one of the largest organs in the body. It has two lobes and fills the upper right side of the abdomen inside the ribcage. The main functions of the liver include the following: to make bile to help digest fat that comes from food, to store glycogen (sugar), which the body uses for energy, and to filter harmful substances from the blood so they can be passed from the body in stools and urine.

Types of liver cancer

Hepatocellular carcinoma (HCC) and bile duct cancer (cholangiocarcinoma) are the main types of adult primary liver cancer.

Most adult primary liver cancers are hepatocellular carcinomas. This type of liver cancer is the third leading cause of cancer-related deaths worldwide.

Primary liver cancer can occur in both adults and children. However, treatment for children is different from treatment for adults.

Signs and symptoms of liver cancer

These and other signs and symptoms may be caused by adult primary liver cancer or by other conditions. Check with your doctor if you have any of the following:

- a hard lump on the right side just below the ribcage
- discomfort in the upper abdomen on the right side
- a swollen abdomen
- pain near the right shoulder blade or in the back
- jaundice (yellowing of the skin and whites of the eyes)
- easy bruising or bleeding
- unusual tiredness or weakness
- nausea and vomiting
- loss of appetite or feelings of fullness after eating a small meal
- weight loss for no known reason
- pale, chalky bowel movements and dark urine
- fever

Causes and risk factors

The most common type of liver cancer in adults, HCC, typically develops in people with chronic (long-lasting) liver disease caused by hepatitis virus infection or cirrhosis. Men are more likely to develop HCC than women. People with multiple risk factors have an even higher risk.

Many risk factors have been associated with liver cancer. Not everyone with one or more of these risk factors will develop the disease, and the disease will develop in some people who don't have any known risk factors. Risk factors include the following.

Hepatitis B virus (HBV) infection

Hepatitis B virus (HBV) can be transmitted in blood, semen, or other body fluids. The infection can be passed from mother to child during childbirth, through sexual contact, or by sharing needles that are used to inject drugs. It can cause inflammation (swelling) of the liver that leads to cancer. Routine HBV vaccination in infancy is reducing the incidence of HBV infection. Chronic HBV infection is the leading cause of liver cancer in Asia and Africa.

Hepatitis C virus (HCV) infection

Hepatitis C virus (HCV) can be transmitted in the blood. The infection can be spread by sharing needles that are used to inject drugs or, less often, through sexual contact. In the past, it was also spread during blood transfusions or organ transplants. Today, blood banks test all donated blood for HCV, which greatly lowers the risk of getting the virus from blood transfusions. It can cause cirrhosis that may lead to liver cancer. Chronic HCV infection is the leading cause of liver cancer in North America, Europe, and Japan.

Cirrhosis

The risk of developing liver cancer is increased for people who have cirrhosis, a disease in which healthy liver tissue is replaced by scar tissue. The scar tissue blocks the flow of blood through the liver and keeps it from working as it should. Chronic alcoholism and chronic hepatitis infections are common causes of cirrhosis. People with HCV-related cirrhosis have a higher risk of developing liver cancer than people with cirrhosis related to HBV or alcohol use.

Heavy alcohol use

Heavy alcohol use can cause cirrhosis, which is a risk factor for liver cancer. Liver cancer can also occur in heavy alcohol users who do not have cirrhosis. Heavy alcohol users who have cirrhosis are ten times more likely to develop liver cancer, compared with heavy alcohol users who do not have cirrhosis.

Studies have shown there is also an increased risk of liver cancer in people with HBV or HCV infection who use alcohol heavily.

Aflatoxin B1

The risk of developing liver cancer may be increased by eating foods that contain aflatoxin B1 (poison from a fungus that can grow on foods, such as corn and nuts, that have been stored in hot, humid places). It is most common in sub-Saharan Africa and Southeast Asia.

Non-alcoholic steatohepatitis (NASH)

Non-alcoholic steatohepatitis (NASH) is a condition that can cause cirrhosis that may lead to liver cancer. It is the most severe form of nonalcoholic fatty liver disease, where there is an abnormal amount of fat in the liver. In some people, this can cause inflammation and injury to the cells of the liver.

Having NASH-related cirrhosis increases the risk of developing liver cancer. Liver cancer has also been found in people with NASH who do not have cirrhosis.

Cigarette smoking

Cigarette smoking has been linked to a higher risk of liver cancer. The risk increases with the number of cigarettes smoked per day and the number of years the person has smoked.

Other conditions

Certain rare medical and genetic conditions may increase the risk of liver cancer. These conditions include untreated hereditary hemochromatosis, alpha-1 antitrypsin deficiency, glycogen storage disease, porphyria cutanea tarda, **and** Wilson's disease.

Types of treatment

Surveillance

Surveillance is used for lesions smaller than 1 centimeter found during screening. Follow-up every 3 months is common. Surveillance is closely watching a patient's condition but not giving any treatment unless there are changes in test results that show the condition is getting worse. During active surveillance, certain exams and tests are done on a regular schedule.

Surgery

A partial hepatectomy (surgery to remove the part of the liver where cancer is found) may be done. A wedge of tissue, an entire lobe, or a larger part of the liver, along with some of the healthy tissue around it is removed. The remaining liver tissue takes over the functions of the liver and may regrow.

Liver transplant

In a liver transplant, the entire liver is removed and replaced with a healthy donated liver. A liver transplant may be done when the disease is in the liver only and a donated liver can be found. If the patient has to wait for a donated liver, other treatment is given as needed.

Ablation therapy

Ablation therapy removes or destroys tissue. Different types of ablation therapy are used for liver cancer:

• Radiofrequency ablation: Special needles are inserted directly through the skin or through an incision in the abdomen to reach the tumor. High-energy radio waves heat the needles and tumor which kills cancer cells.

• Microwave therapy: The tumor is exposed to high temperatures created by microwaves. This can damage and kill cancer cells or make them more sensitive to the effects of radiation and certain anticancer drugs.

• Percutaneous ethanol injection: A small needle is used to inject ethanol (pure alcohol) directly into a tumor to kill cancer cells. Several treatments may be needed. Usually local anesthesia is used, but if the patient has many tumors in the liver, general anesthesia may be used.

• Cryoablation: An instrument is used to freeze and destroy cancer cells. This type of treatment is also called cryotherapy and cryosurgery. The doctor may use ultrasound to guide the instrument.

• Electroporation therapy: Electrical pulses are sent through an electrode placed in a tumor to kill cancer cells. Electroporation therapy is being studied in clinical trials.

Embolization therapy

Embolization therapy is used for patients who cannot have surgery to remove the tumor or ablation therapy and whose tumor has not spread outside the liver. Embolization therapy is the use of substances to block or decrease the flow of blood through the hepatic artery to the tumor. When the tumor does not get the oxygen and nutrients it needs, it will not continue to grow.

The liver receives blood from the hepatic portal vein and the hepatic artery. Blood that comes into the liver from the hepatic portal vein usually goes to the healthy liver tissue. Blood that comes from the hepatic artery usually goes to the tumor. When the hepatic artery is blocked during embolization therapy, the healthy liver tissue continues to receive blood from the hepatic portal vein.

Targeted therapy

Targeted therapy is a type of treatment that uses drugs or other substances to identify and attack specific cancer cells. Targeted therapies usually cause less harm to normal cells than chemotherapy or radiation therapy do.

Immunotherapy

Immunotherapy is a treatment that uses the patient's immune system to fight cancer. Substances made by the body or made in a laboratory are used to boost, direct, or restore the body's natural defenses against cancer.

Radiation therapy

External radiation therapy uses a machine outside the body to send high-energy X-rays or other types of radiation toward the area of the body with cancer. This kills cancer cells or keeps them from growing.

Liver cancer prevention

Cancer prevention is action taken to lower the chance of getting cancer. By preventing cancer, the number of new cases of cancer in a group or population is lowered. Hopefully, this will lower the number of deaths caused by cancer.

Anything that increases your chance of getting cancer is called a risk factor. Anything that lowers your chance of getting cancer is called a cancer protective factor. Prevention includes avoiding risk factors and increasing protective factors.

Protective factors for liver cancer

Getting the hepatitis B vaccine: Preventing HBV infection (by being vaccinated for HBV as a newborn) has been shown to lower the risk of liver cancer in children. It is not yet known if being vaccinated lowers the risk of liver cancer in adults.

Getting treatment for chronic hepatitis B infection: Treatment options for people with chronic HBV infection include interferon and nucleoside (or nucleotide) analog therapy. These treatments may reduce the risk of developing liver cancer.

Reducing exposure to aflatoxin B1: Replacing foods that contain high amounts of aflatoxin B1 with foods that contain a much lower level of the poison can reduce the risk of liver cancer.

It is normal to feel depressed, anxious, or worried when liver cancer is a part of your life. Some people are affected more than others. But everyone can benefit from help and support from other people, whether friends and family, support groups, professional counselors, or others.

(1,763 words)

Task 1

Read the passage above and answer the following questions.

(1) What is primary liver cancer?

(2) What are the main functions of the liver?

(3) What are the main types of adult primary liver cancer?

(4) Can you list some signs and symptoms of liver cancer?

(5) What would typically develop into HCC in adults?

(6) What are the possible risk factors in developing liver cancer?

(7) What types of treatment can be adopted in liver cancer?

(8) In what case the treatment type of surveillance can be taken? And how often should it be conducted?

(9) Which therapy for liver cancer is still being studied in clinic?

(10) Which therapy can be used for patients who cannot have surgery to remove the tumor or ablation therapy and whose tumor has not spread outside the liver?

(11) Which therapy usually causes less harm to normal cells than chemotherapy or radiation therapy do? And why?

(12) What vaccine can be used to prevent people away from liver cancer?

(13) What actions can be taken to prevent people away from liver cancer except for vaccine?

(14) Where can patients with liver cancer get help and support?

Task 2

Read the following paragraph carefully and fill in the blanks with words from the box.

challenging	possible	infections	combination	checkups
exact	depends	trials	exam	removing

Hepatocellular carcinoma (HCC) is a type of liver cancer. It is the second most common liver cancer in children. Doctors don't know the (1) _____ cause of HCC. Children who have viral (2) _____ or other conditions that cause liver inflammation (swelling and irritation), like viral hepatitis, get HCC more often than other children. When a child has HCC, the doctor will do a(n) (3) _____. Tests done may include blood tests, including liver and kidney function tests and an alpha fetoprotein (AFP) test (liver damage and some cancers can raise the level of this protein in the blood); imaging tests, including ultrasound, X-rays, CAT scan and MRI; a biopsy, (4) _____ a piece of tumor tissue for examination or testing. Doctors usually treat HCC with a(n) (5) _____ of surgery and chemotherapy. If (6) _____, children with cancer should go to a medical center specializing in the treatment of pediatric cancers. Treatment (7) _____ on the child's age, the size of the tumor, whether there is one or many tumors in the liver, and whether the cancer has spread from the liver. HCC is (8) _____ to treat, even before it spreads beyond the liver. Clinical (9) _____ are underway to help find better treatments in children and adults. After treatment, a child will have frequent (10) _____ with the care team especially because there is a possibility that the cancer may return.

Task 3

Study the boldfaced words in each of the following sentences and make a sentence of your own.

(1) Primary liver cancer can **occur in** both adults and children.

Your sentence: Liver cancer can also **occur in** heavy alcohol users who do not have cirrhosis.

(2) Many risk factors have **been associated with** liver cancer.

Your sentence: _____

_____

(3) Routine HBV vaccination in infancy is **reducing the incidence of** HBV infection.

Your sentence: _____

_____

(4) The risk of developing liver cancer is increased for people who have cirrhosis, a disease in which healthy liver tissue **is replaced by** scar tissue.

Your sentence: _____

_____

(5) During active surveillance, certain exams and tests are done **on a regular schedule**.

Your sentence: _____

_____

(6) This can damage and kill cancer cells or make them more **sensitive to** the effects of radiation and certain anticancer drugs.

Your sentence: _____

_____

Task 4

Reorder the following sentences into a reasonable paragraph.

(1) In 2005, as the pioneer and trailblazer of China's hepatobiliary surgery, Wu was awarded the State Preeminent Science and Technology Award, China's highest academic accolade.

(2) In 1963, he performed the world's first mesohepatectomy and pushed China to the forefront of liver and gallbladder surgery in the world.

(3) In 1959, Wu's team created the classical liver anatomy theory of "five lobes and four segments," laying the theoretical foundation for China's liver surgery.

(4) In January 2019, the 97-year-old Wu retired in honor and glory. Over his professional career lasting more than 70 years, he saved tens of thousands of patients from the brink of death.

(5) Wu Mengchao, world-famous Chinese hepatobiliary surgery scientist and surgeon, was born in 1922 in a poor family in Fujian Province, and migrated to Malaysia with his family when he was five years old.

(6) In 1940s, he came back to China and was admitted by Tongji University School of Medicine in Shanghai, studying from Qiu Fazu, "father of surgery in China."

Correct order: ____ ____ ____ ____ ____ ____

Story sharing

The following story[①] shares the author's personal experiences as a doctor for Mr. Cheng, who was diagnosed with advanced liver cancer. He tries his best to offer comfort to Mr. Cheng during his last days. Please read the story and finish the tasks.

It was the second time during this frigid December that the elderly Mr. Cheng was found lethargic by his son. Last week, he had injected too much insulin for his diabetes. This week, he'd omitted a dose of his lactulose for the cirrhosis from his advanced liver cancer. Each time, the emergency medical technicians (EMTs) treated Mr. Cheng in the ambulance, so by

---

① Adapted from "The Little Things." Ofri, D. (2014). *New England Journal of Medicine*, 371(15), 1378-1379.

the time we saw him in the emergency room (ER), he was already awake and cantankerous, itching to be discharged. He was fretfully anxious to leave immediately so he wouldn't miss his afternoon dialysis appointment in Chinatown. And he needed his morning dose of Nepro— the nutritional milkshake for dialysis patients.

"He's totally independent," the son told me. "He takes his meds, gets to his appointments, never misses dialysis. The home attendant does cooking and cleaning in the mornings."

But two admissions in 2 weeks for medication errors was a blazing red flag. A frail, elderly man with complicated illnesses, taking high-risk medications, living alone—it was a recipe for disaster.

"Trust me," the son said with a tired smile, "he does not want to be in a nursing home." Mr. Cheng broke in, shaking his rail-thin arms vehemently.

"No nursing home," he said, in his smattering of English. "I go home!"

The social worker applied for increased home-attendant hours. Although the attendant couldn't administer meds, she could remind him to take them. It wasn't ideal, but at least Mr. Cheng was amenable. The catch was that it would take several days for the paperwork to go through, and Mr. Cheng would have to stay in the hospital until then.

"As long as he gets his Nepro," the son said wearily. "He swears by that stuff."

"Nepro," Mr. Cheng echoed, nodding heartily. "Nepro."

And so Mr. Cheng settled into our ward, even though he wasn't acutely ill. He was charming, if a bit ornery, shuffling along the halls to the vending machine. He spoke enough English to greet everyone—and to request his daily Nepro shake. For some reason, although the ward always had a sufficient supply of other nutritional supplements, there never seemed to be much of the kidney version. Our constant requests for stat doses of Nepro on 17-West became a running joke.

Unfortunately for Mr. Cheng, his hospital stay included Christmas, which slowed the already glacial pace of his paperwork.

Every time I had a new patient waiting hours in the ER for a bed, I felt guilty that Mr. Cheng was still in the hospital despite being medically stable. But we were told, "That's the way the system works."

Hospitals are, of course, the worst places for elderly patients, and Mr. Cheng duly illustrated that maxim. Three days into his stay, he spiked a fever, raising concern about peritonitis. We stuck a needle in his swollen belly to check the ascites fluid for infection, but that dropped his hematocrit, so we had to get a CT scan to evaluate the bleed. Mr. Cheng, annoyed by all the procedures, refused his lactulose. That caused him to become lethargic, nearly unresponsive, which, in turn, triggered a "rapid response" of the resuscitation team. His cirrhosis caused his blood pressure to fall, which meant he couldn't get dialysis. Lack of dialysis caused electrolyte chaos.

We finally called a family meeting that Friday morning. Mr. Cheng already knew that his advanced liver cancer gave him a life expectancy in the range of months. But if he couldn't get dialysis, he wouldn't survive more than a week. He signed a DNR form and told us he wanted to go home. Right now.

We protested—the home attendant couldn't come on the weekend. However, Mr. Cheng was adamant. He didn't care about home attendants or hospital protocols. But he did want to be sure we could get his Nepro.

Since he had sufficient decisional capacity, we reluctantly started the discharge process—always a nightmare on a Friday afternoon, especially the one between Christmas and New Year's. When I handed the social worker the inch-thick stack of forms, she tugged out the Nepro prescription and uttered those four dreaded words: "This needs prior authorization."

The prior-authorization process required wading through a tortuous phone tree, punching in everything from the patient's body mass index to his Zodiac sign, and then begging for clemency from a rep whose medical knowledge was probably as limited as Mr. Cheng's remaining kidney function. I knew when I was beaten.

Just then, a supply cart came wheeling around the corner. There on the bottom rack was a glistening case of Nepro shakes. I looked from the cart to the nurse, social worker, resident, and intern. "Maybe I'll just lift a few of these," I joked, and everyone chuckled. It would certainly be more efficient than battling Medicaid for prior authorization on the eve of a 3-day holiday weekend.

I flashed my most ingratiating smile at the orderly. "Would you mind if I just grabbed one of those Nepro shakes?" The orderly froze me with a granite institutional stare.

"Please," I said, "it's for one of our patients." I didn't mention that I was planning to abet the patient in smuggling them out of the hospital—a flagrant violation of inpatient-outpatient turf boundaries. The orderly hesitated but then gave a grudging nod. I pulled two cans from the cart and stuffed them into the pockets of my white coat.

Then I thought about the upcoming weekend. Mr. Cheng would be alone, and Nepro seemed to be the only thing that brought him pleasure. When the orderly turned to stock the supply cabinet, I whisked out two more cans, tucking them under the discharge papers.

Monday was a holiday, too—3 long days for Mr. Cheng, maybe his final days. I snagged two more cans and rolled them in the medical journal I was carrying.

What if he woke up at night, hungry? I grabbed another two and jammed them under my crossed arms.

When the orderly finally rolled his cart away, I turned toward my team and nodded. "I believe we have Mr. Cheng's discharge plan in order."

I went to Mr. Cheng and told him he was going home. "The Nepro?" he asked anxiously. I plopped a bag of the pilfered Nepro at his bedside. His face lit up, his eyes crinkling from the effort of containing his radiant grin. I shook his hand good-bye and wished him well.

Two hours later, the authorization for the ambulette came through. The nurse who'd gone into Mr. Cheng's room to give him his discharge papers suddenly came dashing out. "He's ... he's passed," she said, breathlessly. "Mr. Cheng has died."

We followed her into the room, and there was Mr. Cheng—face calm, body still. We quietly verified the absence of respirations and pulse and then stood in a semicircle around his bed.

By all appearances he'd died peacefully. We were glad for that, but he hadn't gotten his fervent wish to be at home. At the bedside was his bag of precious Nepro cans—pristine, unopened.

We stood together in a moment of contemplative silence. Then the son grabbed the bag of Nepro and pressed it to me. "We won't be needing this now," he said with a rueful smile. I took the bag, and our hands briefly closed over each other's.

For the next 2 weeks, the bag sat under my desk; I couldn't bear to return the Nepro. There was something achingly poignant about these little cans that had meant so much to Mr. Cheng.

For patients like Mr. Cheng, we rightly try to focus on the big picture, rather than the nitty-gritty of prodding potassium or nudging glucose. But sometimes, amidst the collapsing dominoes of relentless illness, it's the little picture that makes the most palpable difference. The assurance that his Nepro would be there appeared to give Mr. Cheng more comfort than anything else we could offer.

(1,321 words)

Task 1

Read the passage above and write a paragraph to complete it, with the first sentence being provided.

Many patients have their own versions of Mr. Cheng's Nepro.

_____

_____

_____

_____

_____

_____

_____

Task 2

Discuss the following questions in groups.

(1) What is the Nepro in Mr. Cheng's eyes?

(2) What lessons can you learn from the author's role as a doctor?

(3) What lessons can you learn from Mr. Cheng?

Vocabulary checklist

英文	中文
* **digestive** system [daɪˈdʒestɪv]	消化系统
* salivate [ˈsælɪveɪt]	分泌唾液
feces [ˈfiːsiːz]	粪便
* anus [ˈeɪnəs]	肛门
amino acid [əˈmiːnəʊ]	氨基酸
starch [ˈstɑːtʃ]	淀粉;含淀粉的食物
fatty acid	脂肪酸
glycerol [ˈɡlɪsərɒl]	甘油
alimentary canal [ˌælɪˈmentəri kəˈnæl]	消化管
* pancreas [ˈpæŋkriəs]	胰腺
* esophagus [ɪˈsɒfəɡəs]	食管
intestine [ɪnˈtestɪn]	肠

英文	中文
* salivary gland [səˈlaɪvəri glænd]	唾液腺
* enzyme [ˈenzaɪm]	酶
amylase [ˈæmɪleɪz]	淀粉酶
carbohydrate [ˌkɑːbəʊˈhaɪdreɪt]	碳水化合物
* pharynx [ˈfærɪŋks]	咽
epiglottis [ˌepɪˈglɒtɪs]	会厌
* peristalsis [ˌperɪˈstælsɪs]	蠕动
sphincter [ˈsfɪŋktə(r)]	括约肌
chyme [kaɪm]	食糜
pylorus [paɪˈlɔːrəs]	幽门
* duodenum [ˌdjuːəˈdiːnəm]	十二指肠
jejunum [dʒɪˈdʒuːnəm]	空肠
ileum [ˈɪliəm]	回肠
villi [ˈvɪlaɪ]	绒毛(villus 的复数)
ribcage [ˈrɪbkeɪdʒ]	胸腔
* abdomen [ˈæbdəmən]	腹部
* gall bladder	胆囊

英文	中文
＊ bile ［baɪl］	胆汁
carbs	碳水化合物
duct ［dʌkt］	输送管
excrete ［ɪkˈskriːt］	排泄
＊ cecum ［ˈsiːkəm］	盲肠
＊ colon ［ˈkəʊlən］	结肠
＊ rectum ［ˈrektəm］	直肠
ascending colon	升结肠
transverse colon	横结肠
descending colon	降结肠
sigmoid colon ［ˈsɪɡmɒɪd］	乙状结肠
bowel movement ［ˈbaʊəl］	排便
＊ primary liver cancer	原发性肝癌
malignant（cancer）cell ［məˈlɪɡnənt］	恶性肿瘤（癌）细胞
lobe ［ləʊb］	瓣
glycogen ［ˈɡlaɪkədʒən］	糖原
＊ stool ［stuːl］	大便
hepatocellular carcinoma ［ˌhepətəʊˈseljʊlə ˌkɑːsɪˈnəʊmə］	肝细胞癌
bile duct cancer	胆管癌

英文	中文
cholangiocarcinoma [kəʊlədʒiːəʊkɑːsɪˈnəʊmə]	胆管细胞癌
signs and symptoms	病征与症状
shoulder blade	肩胛骨
* jaundice [ˈdʒɔːndɪs]	黄疸
nausea [ˈnɔːziə]	恶心
vomit	呕吐
* **hepatitis** virus [ˌhepəˈtaɪtɪs]	肝炎病毒
* cirrhosis [səˈrəʊsɪs]	肝硬化
hepatitis B virus	乙型肝炎病毒
semen [ˈsiːmən]	精液
hepatitis C virus	丙型肝炎病毒
blood transfusion	输血
scar tissue	瘢痕组织
alcoholism [ˈælkəhɒlɪzəm]	酗酒
aflatoxin B1 [ˌæfləˈtɒksɪn]	黄曲霉毒素 B1
fungus [ˈfʌŋgəs]	真菌
non-alcoholic **steatohepatitis** [ˌstiətəʊhepəˈtaɪtɪs]	非酒精性脂肪性肝炎
hereditary hemochromatosis [həˈredɪtri ˌhiːməʊkrəʊməˈtəʊsɪs]	遗传性血色病
alpha-1 **antitrypsin** deficiency [ˌæntɪˈtrɪpsɪn]	α1-抗胰蛋白酶缺乏症

英文	中文
glycogen storage disease	糖原贮积症
porphyria cutanea tarda [pɔːˈfɪrɪə kʊˈteɪnɪə ˈtɑːdə]	迟发性皮肤卟啉病
Wilson's disease	肝豆状核变性,威尔逊氏症
* lesion [ˈliːʒn]	病变
hepatectomy [ˌhepəˈtektəmi]	肝切除术
ablation therapy [əˈbleɪʃn]	消融疗法
radiofrequency ablation [ˌreɪdɪəʊˈfriːkwənsi]	射频消融术
incision [ɪnˈsɪʒn]	切口
percutaneous ethanol injection [ˌpɜːkjuːˈteɪnɪəs] [ˈeθənɒl]	经皮乙醇注射治疗
* local **anesthesia** [ˌænəsˈθiːzɪə]	局部麻醉
* general anesthesia	全身麻醉
cryoablation [kraɪəʊəbˈleɪʃən]	冷冻消融(术)
electroporation therapy [ɪˌlektrəʊpɔːˈreɪʃn]	电穿孔疗法
electrical pulse	电脉冲
electrode [ɪˈlektrəʊd]	电极
embolization therapy [embəlaɪˈzeɪʃən]	栓塞疗法
hepatic artery [hɪˈpætɪk ˈɑːtəri]	肝动脉
hepatic **portal vein** [ˈpɔːtl] [veɪn]	肝门静脉

英文	中文
targeted therapy	靶向治疗
immunotherapy [ˌɪmjʊˈnəʊˈθerəpi]	免疫疗法
radiation therapy	放射疗法
nucleoside analog therapy [ˈnjuːkliəsaɪd] [ˈænəlɒɡ]	核苷模拟疗法
lethargic [ləˈθɑːdʒɪk]	昏睡的
insulin [ˈɪnsjəlɪn]	胰岛素
lactulose [ˌlæktʊˈləʊz]	乳果糖
dialysis [ˌdaɪˈæləsɪs]	透析
peritonitis [ˌperɪtəˈnaɪtɪs]	腹膜炎
ascites fluid [əˈsaɪtiːz]	腹水
hematocrit [ˈhemətəʊkrɪt]	红细胞比容
electrolyte [ɪˈlektrəlaɪt]	电解质
body mass index	体重指数
ambulette [ˈæmbjʊlet]	轻型救护车
* respiration [ˌrespəˈreɪʃn]	呼吸
potassium [pəˈtæsiəm]	钾
* glucose [ˈgluːkəʊs]	葡萄糖

注：＊表示高频医学英语词汇。

Urinary system

Upon completion of this chapter, you will be able to

❖ name the parts of the urinary system and the structures that transport and store urine;

❖ describe the functions of the urinary system;

❖ list major pathologic conditions affecting the urinary system;

❖ understand information about chronic kidney diseases;

❖ gather information about common urinary diseases;

❖ present one common urinary disease with group members.

Theme reading 1

An introduction to the urinary tract[1]

What is the urinary tract?

The urinary tract is one of the systems that our bodies use to get rid of waste products. The kidneys are the part of the urinary tract that makes urine (pee). Urine has salts, toxins, and water that need to be filtered out of the blood. After the kidneys make urine, it leaves the body using the rest of the urinary tract as a pathway.

What are the parts of the urinary tract?

People usually have two kidneys, but can live a normal, healthy life with just one. The kidneys are under the ribcage in the back, one on each side. Each adult kidney is about the size of a fist.

Each kidney has an outer layer called the cortex, which contains filtering units. The center part of the kidney, the medulla, has fan-shaped structures called pyramids. These

---

① Adapted from "Kidneys and Urinary Tract." Hirsch, L. (2018). https://kidshealth.org

drain urine into cup-shaped tubes called calyxes.

From the calyxes, pee travels out of the kidneys through the ureters to be stored in the bladder (a muscular sac in the lower belly). When a person urinates, the pee exits the bladder and goes out of the body through the urethra, another tube-like structure. The male urethra ends at the tip of the penis; the female urethra ends just above the vaginal opening.

What do the kidneys do?

Kidneys have many jobs, from filtering blood and making pee to keeping bones healthy and making a hormone that controls the production of red blood cells.

The kidneys also help regulate blood pressure, the level of salts in the blood, and the acid-base balance (the pH) of the blood. All these jobs make the kidneys essential to keeping the body working as it should.

How does the urinary tract work?

Blood travels to each kidney through the renal artery. The artery enters the kidney at the hilum, the indentation in middle of the kidney that gives it its bean shape. The artery then branches so blood can get to the nephrons—1 million tiny filtering units in each kidney that remove the harmful substances from the blood.

Each of the nephrons contain a filter called the glomerulus. The fluid that is filtered out from the blood then travels down a tiny tube-like structure called a tubule. The tubule adjusts the level of salts, water, and wastes that will leave the body in the urine. Filtered blood leaves the kidney through the renal vein and flows back to the heart.

Pee leaves the kidneys and travels through the ureters to the bladder. The bladder expands as it fills. When the bladder is full, nerve endings in its wall send messages to the brain. When a person needs to pee, the bladder walls tighten and a ring-like muscle that guards the exit from the bladder to the urethra, called the sphincter, relaxes. This lets pee go into the urethra and out of the body.

How can I keep my urinary tract healthy?

Here are some ways to help keep your kidneys and urinary tract healthy:

- Get plenty of exercise.
- Eat a nutritious diet.
- Stay hydrated.
- For girls: Wipe from front to back after pooping so germs don't get into the urethra.
- Avoid bubble baths, sitting in the tub after shampoo has been used, and scented soaps. These can irritate the urethra.
- Wear cotton underwear.
- Promptly change out of wet bathing suits.
- Go for regular medical checkups.
- Talk to your doctor before taking any supplements or herbal treatments.
- Let the doctor know about any family history of kidney problems, diabetes, or high

blood pressure.

- Let the doctor know if you have any swelling or puffiness, have pain with peeing, need to pee often, have foamy urine or blood in the urine, or are constipated.

(635 words)

Task 1

Read the passage above and answer the following questions.

(1) What is the urinary tract?

(2) What are the parts of the urinary tract?

(3) What do the kidneys do?

(4) How does the urinary tract work?

(5) What ways can keep your urinary tract healthy?

Task 2

Please label Figure 4-1 and Figure 4-2 with the medical terms you've learnt in Theme reading 1.

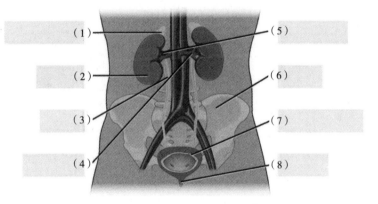

Figure 4-1   Urinary system[①]

(1) adrenal gland	(2)
(3)	(4) renal vein
(5) renal artery	(6) pelvis
(7)	(8)

---

① Adapted from "Urinary system anatomy and physiology." Belleza, M. (2021) https://nurseslabs.com

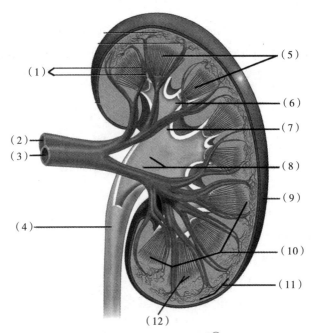

Figure 4-2　The kidney[①]

(1) interlobar arteries and veins	(2) renal artery
(3) renal vein	(4)
(5) renal pyramids	(6) minor calyx
(7) major calyx	(8) renal pelvis
(9)	(10) medulla
(11)	(12) nephrons

① Adapted from "Label the kidney" (n. d.). https://anatomycorner.com

Task 3

Figure 4-3 shows how the kidneys work. Please describe each step by one or two sentences and write them down on the blanks below the figure.

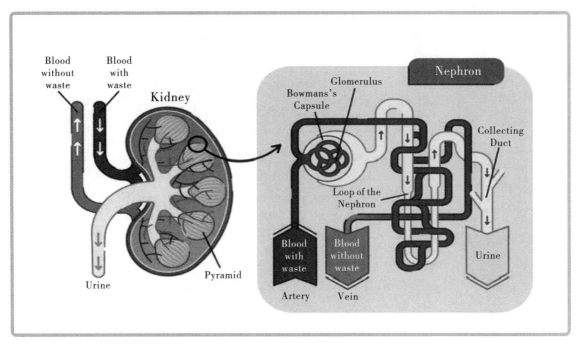

Figure 4-3   How the kidneys work[①]

(1)

(2)

(3)

(4)

Vocabulary bridge

Study the following terms for common signs, symptoms and diseases related to the urinary system and translate them into Chinese.

Medical terms	Explanation	Chinese translations
azoturia	increase of nitrogenous substances, especially urea, in urine	氮尿症

① Adapted from "Kidney functionality, diseases and treatment options" (n. d.). https://kidneyurology.org

Medical terms	Explanation	Chinese translations
diuresis	increased formation and secretion of urine	
dysuria	painful or difficult urination, symptomatic of cystitis and other urinary tract conditions	
end-stage renal disease	kidney disease that has advanced to the point that the kidneys can no longer adequately filter the blood and, ultimately, requires dialysis or renal transplantation for survival	
enuresis	involuntary discharge of urine after the age at which bladder control should be established	
hypospadias	abnormal congenital opening of the male urethra on the undersurface of the penis	
interstitial nephritis	condition associated with pathological changes in the renal interstitial tissue that may be primary or due to a toxic agent, such as a drug or chemical, which results in destruction of nephrons and severe impairment in renal function	
renal hypertension	high blood pressure that results from kidney disease	
uremia	elevated level of urea and other nitrogenous waste products in the blood, as occurs in renal failure; also called azotemia	
Wilms tumor	malignant neoplasm of the kidney that occurs in young children, usually before age 5	

Theme reading 2

Chronic kidney disease[①]

What is chronic kidney disease?

Chronic kidney disease (CKD) means that your kidneys do not work as well as they should. They can't remove waste products from your body. Damage to the kidney's filter system can also allow blood and protein to leak into the urine. This is not always visible but can be found with a urine test.

The term "chronic" means that it is a long-term condition. It does not necessarily mean your kidney damage is severe as many cases of CKD are mild and can be managed with help from your GP (general practitioner) and without hospital involvement.

How is CKD diagnosed?

Most people are diagnosed by a blood and urine test. You may have these tests as part of

---

① Adapted from "Chronic kidney disease (CKD)" (n.d.). https://www.kidneycareuk.org

a routine check-up or because you are at risk of developing CKD.

Once you are diagnosed, your doctor will work out what stage of CKD you have (see Table 4-1). This is done by measuring the amount of creatinine, a waste product which builds up in kidney disease. Your doctors can use this to estimate how well your kidneys are working. You may hear this referred to as your estimated glomerular filtration rate (e-GFR). It is based on how quickly your kidneys are cleaning your blood and is measured in millilitres per minute.

Table 4-1　Stages of chronic kidney disease

Stage	Description	e-GFR Level
One	Kidney function remains normal but urine findings suggest kidney disease	90 ml/min or more
Two	Slightly reduced kidney function with urine findings suggesting kidney disease	60 to 89 ml/min
Three	Moderately reduced kidney function	30 to 59 ml/min
Four	Severely reduced kidney function	15 to 29 ml/min
Five	Very severe or end-stage kidney failure	Less than 15 ml/min or on dialysis

CKD can slowly get worse over time, although for the majority of people it remains stable and only a very small number of people will need renal replacement therapy such as dialysis. It is unusual for kidney function to improve dramatically once your kidneys have been damaged but it does depend on the cause of the problem.

Causes

There are lots of causes of CKD. The most common causes include diabetes, heart disease, high blood pressure (hypertension), inflammation within the kidneys (glomerulonephritis), blockages to the flow of urine such as prostate problems or cancers in the bladder, certain medications such as non-steroidal anti-inflammatory drugs (NSAIDs) which include ibuprofen (Brufen or Nurofen) or diclofenac (Voltarol) among others, and family history of kidney disease which may include inherited diseases.

Signs and symptoms

Most people do not have symptoms related to CKD. Even when your kidneys are damaged, they can still work well enough to prevent you having any symptoms. You can be born with just the one kidney and remain healthy.

You may still produce normal amounts of urine, even if you have CKD, but your kidneys are unable to remove the toxins from your body that they need to in order to keep you healthy. It is the quality rather than quantity of urine that you produce that matters.

Symptoms may only be noticeable with more advanced kidney disease. These include generally feeling ill, lack of interest in everyday activities, loss of concentration, tiredness, low energy levels, muscle weakness, finding it difficult to breathe (due to a build-up of fluid in the lungs), difficulty sleeping at night (insomnia), passing urine more often at night, feeling sick, headaches, itching, aching bones, and muscle cramps.

For most people with chronic kidney disease there is only a mild or moderate reduction in kidney function with few symptoms. However, it can develop to a more serious stage where the kidneys no longer work—this is called kidney failure.

Around 10% of people with CKD may reach a stage that is known as established renal failure when the kidneys can no longer work well enough to keep us healthy and alive, and support from dialysis treatment or a kidney transplant is considered.

Why does it matter if I have CKD and don't have any symptoms?

Although you may not have any symptoms from CKD, kidney damage can still affect your health. CKD can increase your chance of having high blood pressure, heart disease or a stroke. It is therefore important that you are reviewed regularly by either your GP or your kidney doctor.

Having CKD gives you a higher risk of developing acute kidney injury (AKI). This is a sudden drop in kidney function, often due to an illness or infection. AKI can usually be treated very effectively but it can cause a permanent reduction in your kidney function.

Treatment choices

Dialysis is an artificial way of removing waste products and unwanted water from your blood. You can choose between haemodialysis and peritoneal dialysis.

During haemodialysis, blood flows out of your body, round a dialysis machine, through a dialyser (artificial kidney) which cleans it and it is then returned to your body. This can be done at home, in a "satellite" haemodialysis unit near your home, or in a dialysis unit in a main hospital. You will need a small operation to create a "fistula," which is where an artery is joined to a vein, so that the vein can be made bigger to allow dialysis needles to reach your bloodstream. This is usually done six months before you start dialysis, to give it time to enlarge although they can usually be used safely after about six weeks if necessary. If you need dialysis before a fistula is made, you may have a temporary dialysis line (a small plastic tube) put into a large vein in your neck.

During peritoneal dialysis, fluid is passed into your abdomen up to four times a day, or overnight at home. This type of dialysis involves putting a small, soft, plastic tube called a catheter into your abdomen (tummy area), which allows dialysis fluid to be drained in and out of what is called your peritoneal cavity. Waste products are passed from your blood and are absorbed by the dialysis fluid. When the fluid is drained out it takes the waste and extra fluid out of your body.

This can be done either by hand four times a day via a process called CAPD (continuous ambulatory peritoneal dialysis), or by machine overnight and known as APD (automated peritoneal dialysis). CAPD takes about 20 – 30 minutes to drain the fluid in and out and needs to be done four times a day. APD takes place for eight hours overnight and needs 30 minutes to set up and clean the machine before and after each treatment.

Some patients choose a path called conservative treatment rather than treatment with dialysis. This may suit people with other medical conditions who feel dialysis is not for them.

Transplantation is the best treatment for the majority of patients with established renal failure. Transplantation extends life expectancy, improves quality of life and offers freedom from dialysis. This is the most successful treatment for kidney failure. Donated kidneys come from two sources: the national deceased (cadaveric) donor pool or a living donor. Kidneys from living donors offer the best chance of success overall and prevent the need to join the national transplant waiting list.

A kidney transplant before starting dialysis (known as a preemptive transplant) is the gold standard of choice, as patients can avoid the need for dialysis altogether and the kidney is likely to last longer.

Unfortunately, not everyone is suitable for renal transplantation, particularly those with multiple other medical conditions, or people of advanced age. All patients have to have tests to ensure they are fit enough to receive a transplant, and some may need particular medical conditions to be treated, or (in addition) they may need to lose some weight, before they are able to receive a kidney transplant.

Some patients would rather not have any treatment for their kidney failure and many units now have a dedicated team of nurses who are able to provide support and care for these patients and their families. It is important to remember that dialysis and transplantation are not for everyone and that people have the right to choose not to be treated.

(1,290 words)

Task 1

Read the passage above and answer the following questions.

(1) What is chronic kidney disease (CKD)?

(2) How is CKD diagnosed?

(3) How many stages is CKD divided?

(4) What are the causes of CKD?

(5) What are the symptoms of CKD?

(6) What is kidney failure?

(7) How are patients with kidney failure treated?

(8) What is haemodialysis?

(9) What is peritoneal dialysis?

(10) What are the two ways of peritoneal dialysis?

(11) Besides dialysis, what can patients choose?

(12) What are the two sources of kidney transplant?

(13) What do patients need to do before deciding whether they are suitable for kidney transplant?

Task 2

Read the following paragraphs carefully and fill in the blanks with the words from the box.

further	confirm	disease	down	provide
protein	normal	treatment	amount	quick

One of the earliest signs of kidney disease is when (1)_____ leaks into your urine (called proteinuria). To check for protein in your urine, a doctor will order a urine test. There are two types of urine tests that can check your protein levels.

Dipstick urine test is often done as part of an overall urinalysis, but it can also be done as a (2)_____ test to look for albumin (a protein produced by your liver) in your urine. It does not (3)_____ an exact measurement of albumin but does let your doctor know if your levels are normal. A dipstick (a chemically treated paper) is placed in a urine sample you provide and if levels are above (4)_____, the dipstick changes color. If you have abnormal albumin levels, your doctor may want to run (5)_____ tests.

Urine albumin-to-creatinine ratio (UACR) measures the (6)_____ of albumin and compares it to the amount of creatinine (a waste product that comes from the normal wear and tear of muscles in the body) in your urine. A UACR test lets the doctor know how much albumin passes into your urine over a 24-hour period. A urine albumin test result of 30 or above may mean kidney (7)_____.

It's important to know that the test may be repeated once or twice to (8)_____ the results. If you do have kidney disease, the amount of albumin in your urine helps your doctor know which (9)_____ is best for you. A urine albumin level that stays the same or goes (10)_____ means that your treatment is working.

Task 3

Study the boldfaced words in each of the following sentences and make a sentence of your own.

(1) When the fluid is **drained out** it takes the waste and extra fluid out of your body.

Your sentence: About 100 ml of cloudy fluid was **drained out** from the little girl's abdomen.

(2) Patients who choose not to have dialysis are usually managed **in the same way as** other patients with CKD.

Your sentence: _____

_____

(3) Most people do not have symptoms **related to** CKD.

Your sentence: _____

_____

(4) It is the quality **rather than** quantity of urine that you produce that matters.

Your sentence: _____

_____

(5) APD **takes place** for eight hours overnight and needs 30 minutes to set up and clean the machine before and after each treatment.

Your sentence: _____

_____

(6) This is done by measuring the amount of creatinine, a waste product which **builds up** in kidney disease.

Your sentence: _____

_____

Task 4

Reorder the following sentences into a reasonable paragraph.

(1) After that visit, each time you go you will have your weight and blood pressure measured and a sample of your urine will be checked for signs of blood, protein or infection.

(2) You will then speak to the doctor about your symptoms and discuss which treatments are available.

(3) At the first visit, your specialist kidney doctor will try and find out the cause of your CKD.

(4) You will have a blood test to measure your kidney function and check for signs of anemia, bone health and blood acidity levels.

Correct order: ____ ____ ____ ____

Story sharing

The following story① is written by Jennie, a psychotherapeutic counsellor and carer for her husband Geoff, who was diagnosed with CKD in June 2016. She shares her personal experiences as a carer for her husband. Please read the story and finish the tasks.

It's the little things that can affect you most when you are a carer for someone with a chronic illness.

I work as a psychotherapeutic counsellor and am used to supporting others. But I have learned through our experience of CKD how the grueling schedule of daily care can take its toll on the carer.

Small details take over your life. The health service is under-resourced and over-stretched, and can tend to focus on the patient rather than the supporting "home team," who are every bit as important.

When my husband Geoff was diagnosed with CKD in June 2016, we were initially stunned by the diagnosis. An optician identified bleeding behind the retina and referred him to our GP. Our GP then confirmed that Geoff's kidney function was down to 20％. Now we understood Geoff's increasing tiredness and regular chest infections over the winter months. We limped along until September that year when he finally had a peritoneal catheter inserted. At this point his kidney function was just 6％. Geoff spent his days resting on the sofa—not in any discomfort, but quietly "slipping away"—or so it seemed.

However, the catheter insertion gave us new hope. As I was still working, friends kindly helped transport Geoff to and from Norfolk and Norwich hospital. Health personnel came to assess the premises for the automated peritoneal dialysis (APD) machine, and our two sons lugged the massive boxes of dialysis fluid (two bags a night) up our two flights of stairs in our tiny thatched cottage, every evening. I spent many hours on the phone in the middle of the night to the 24-hour help line, and frequently slept in my workroom as the alarms woke me up constantly. Stopping work was not an option, as I am self-employed and we could not pay the mortgage without the income.

We got to a point where the nurses suggested we go on to the day-time bags instead. This at least relieved us of the disturbed nights. But the presence of discarded bags of dialysis fluid left around the living room during the day, began to get to me. One day I had a melt down at the hospital. I could feel my days turning into a constant cycle of clearing up used dialysis bags and living in what was rapidly beginning to resemble a badly run nursing home. At this, Geoff

①Adapted from "Who cares for the carer?." Cummings-Knight, J. (2020). https://www.kidneycareuk.org

who had been quite passive about what was happening to him up to this point, suddenly recognized that I was not coping.

This realization had a profound effect on him and he began to take responsibility for his own care.

It took us about four months to get used to the new routine of daytime bags. At this point it was suggested that Geoff should go on to the transplant waiting list. Talking this through with the consultant, we were given so many warnings about what could potentially go wrong that we were puzzled when he said, "So you are eligible. Isn't that great! Let's go ahead." We mulled it over for a while and decided to wait for six months.

Geoff's transplant took place in April 2018. And the transplant itself went well. But alas, it failed just under a year later. Between February and July 2019 Geoff spent a total of 12 weeks in hospital with a variety of complications. He woke after surgery and was his usual groggy self. Twenty-four hours went by and he was unable to go to pass urine. The doctors said that this could happen after surgery. Thirty-six hours passed and we knew something wasn't right. I called the nurse and told her. Geoff had some symptoms of renal failure and we just knew what was happening. Geoff started to shiver. He was itching, and he was getting cramps. Six months on (currently on haemodialysis), he is now awaiting surgery for the re-insertion of a peritoneal catheter. That one year of freedom was all he had and the chance of a new beginning was snatched from him and us. He was, we all were, so very upset.

However, one thing that helped me during this difficult time was writing poetry. The range of emotions that we feel as a carer needs to be expressed and we sometimes find it difficult to admit just how angry we are at what life has dealt us. Poetry enabled me to express these feelings. By writing poetry, I once again discovered who I really was instead of being overwhelmed by the daily routines. It also helped me stay in tune with my thoughts and feelings. It just functioned as a therapeutic process which was not only healthy for my mind but for the soul as well. As a great outlet to express my negative feelings in a safe way, I sometimes even shared my poems with Geoff. I found they acted as a great way to better connect us.

As a mother of three, I well remember how maternal instincts develop when the first baby comes along—the slightest sound wakes you up and you are intimately attuned to every signal in order to care for that baby and keep it safe. For me, this feeling of hyper-vigilance is once again with me all the time. The moment Geoff voices his discomfort, I'd be very attentive, sometimes even too attentive. After all these years, Geoff becomes my baby.

If any of this resonates with you, I leave you with a question: are you looking after yourself, as well as you look after your loved one? Receiving treatment for CKD is a life-long commitment to some form of renal replacement therapy (RRT). It can be an arduous journey and not many of us travel this journey alone. I definitely would not like you to feel that you are alone on this journey. The diagnosis of CKD affects everyone around us and the impact on our partners, loved ones, and home life can never be underestimated.

(994 words)

Task 1

Read the passage above and write a paragraph to complete it, with the first sentence being provided.

I am so thankful for all the support that I have had from local friends and from family members.

_____

_____

_____

_____

_____

_____

_____

_____

_____

_____

_____

_____

Task 2

Discuss the following questions in groups.

(1) How can we take care of people with CKD? Please give some specific examples.

(2) What factors brought hope to Jennie and made her get through eventually?

(3) When we are having a hard time as carers, what can we do for ourselves?

(4) What lessons can you learn from the author's experience?

Vocabulary checklist

英文	中文
* urinary tract [juərɪnəri trækt]	尿路，泌尿道
* ribcage [ˈrɪbkeɪdʒ]	胸腔
* cortex [ˈkɔːteks]	皮质
* medulla [meˈdʌlə]	髓质
* pyramid [ˈpɪrəmɪd]	肾锥体
calyx [ˈkeɪlɪks]	肾盏
* ureter [juˈriːtə (r)]	输尿管
* bladder [ˈblædə (r)]	膀胱
* urethra [juˈriːθrə]	尿道
vaginal opening [vəˈdʒaɪnl ˈəʊpənɪŋ]	阴道口
acid-base balance [ˈæsɪd]	酸碱平衡
* renal artery [ˈriːnl ˈɑːtəri]	肾动脉
hilum [ˈhaɪləm]	肾门
* nephron [ˈnefrɒn]	肾单位
* glomerulus [gləʊˈmerjʊləs]	肾小球

英文	中文
* tubule [ˈtjuːbjuːl]	肾小管
* renal **vein** [veɪn]	肾静脉
* sphincter [ˈsfɪŋktə (r)]	括约肌
GP (general practitioner)	全科医师
creatinine [krɪˈætɪnɪn]	尿肌酐
glomerular filtration rate [ɡləʊˈmerjʊlə] [fɪlˈtreɪʃn]	肾小球滤过率
glomerulonephritis [ɡləʊˌmerjʊləʊneˈfraɪtɪs]	肾小球肾炎
* prostate [ˈprɒsteɪt]	前列腺
non-**steroidal** anti-**inflammatory** drugs [steˈrɒɪdəl] [ɪnˈflæmətri]	非甾体抗炎药
ibuprofen [ˌaɪbjuːˈprəʊfen]	布洛芬
diclofenac [dɪklɒfeˈnæk]	双氯芬酸
* insomnia [ɪnˈsɒmniə]	失眠
* kidney failure	肾衰竭
* kidney **transplant** [trænsˈplɑːnt]	肾移植
acute kidney injury	急性肾损伤
haemodialysis [ˌhiːməʊdaɪˈæləsɪs]	血液透析
peritoneal dialysis [ˌperɪtəʊˈniːəl ˌdaɪˈæləsɪs]	腹膜透析

英文	中文
dialyser [ˈdaɪəˌlaɪzə]	透析器
fistula [ˈfɪstʃələ]	瘘管
* abdomen [ˈæbdəmən]	腹部
catheter [ˈkæθətə (r)]	导尿管
* peritoneal **cavity** [ˈkævəti]	腹膜腔
CAPD (continuous ambulatory peritoneal dialysis)	持续不卧床腹膜透析
APD (automated peritoneal dialysis)	自动腹膜透析
conservative treatment [kənˈsɜːvətɪv]	保守治疗
retina [ˈretɪnə]	视网膜

注：＊表示高频医学英语词汇。

Reproductive system

Upon completion of this chapter, you will be able to

❖ name major organs of the female and male reproductive system;

❖ describe fertilization process in humans;

❖ list major pathologic conditions affecting the reproductive organs;

❖ understand information about ovarian cancer;

❖ gather information about common disorders affecting the reproductive system;

❖ present one common reproductive system disease with group members.

Theme reading 1

An introduction to the reproductive system[①]

What is reproduction?

Reproduction is the process by which organisms make more organisms like themselves. But even though the reproductive system is essential to keeping a species alive, unlike other body systems, it's not essential to keeping an individual alive.

In the human reproductive process, two kinds of sex cells, or gametes, are involved. The male gamete, or sperm, and the female gamete, the egg or ovum, meet in the female's reproductive system. When sperm fertilizes (meets) an egg, this fertilized egg is called a zygote. The zygote goes through a process of becoming an embryo and developing into a fetus.

The male reproductive system and the female reproductive system both are needed for reproduction. Humans, like other organisms, pass some characteristics of themselves to the

---

① Adapted from "Female & male reproductive System." Hirsch, L. (2018). https://kidshealth.org

next generation. We do this through our genes, the special carriers of human traits. The genes that parents pass along are what make their children similar to others in their family, but also what make each child unique. These genes come from the male's sperm and the female's egg.

What is the female reproductive system?

The external part of the female reproductive organs is called the vulva, which means covering. Located between the legs, the vulva covers the opening to the vagina and other reproductive organs inside the body.

The fleshy area located just above the top of the vaginal opening is called the mons pubis. Two pairs of skin flaps called the labia (which means lips) surround the vaginal opening. The clitoris, a small sensory organ, is located toward the front of the vulva where the folds of the labia join. Between the labia are openings to the urethra (the canal that carries pee from the bladder to the outside of the body) and vagina. When girls become sexually mature, the outer labia and the mons pubis are covered by pubic hair.

A female's internal reproductive organs are the vagina, uterus, fallopian tubes, and ovaries.

The vagina is a muscular, hollow tube that extends from the vaginal opening to the uterus. Because it has muscular walls, the vagina can expand and contract. This ability to become wider or narrower allows the vagina to accommodate something as slim as a tampon and as wide as a baby. The vagina's muscular walls are lined with mucous membranes, which keep it protected and moist.

The vagina connects with the uterus, or womb, at the cervix (which means neck). The cervix has strong, thick walls. The opening of the cervix is very small (no wider than a straw), which is why a tampon can never get lost inside a girl's body. During childbirth, the cervix can expand to allow a baby to pass.

The uterus is shaped like an upside-down pear, with a thick lining and muscular walls— in fact, the uterus contains some of the strongest muscles in the female body. These muscles are able to expand and contract to accommodate a growing fetus and then help push the baby out during labor. When a woman isn't pregnant, the uterus is only about 3 inches (7.5 centimeters) long and 2 inches (5 centimeters) wide.

At the upper corners of the uterus, the fallopian tubes connect the uterus to the ovaries. The ovaries are two oval-shaped organs that lie to the upper right and left of the uterus. They produce, store, and release eggs into the fallopian tubes in the process called ovulation.

There are two fallopian tubes, each attached to a side of the uterus. Within each tube is a tiny passageway no wider than a sewing needle. At the other end of each fallopian tube is a fringed area that looks like a funnel. This fringed area wraps around the ovary but doesn't completely attach to it. When an egg pops out of an ovary, it enters the fallopian tube. Once the egg is in the fallopian tube, tiny hairs in the tube's lining help push it down the narrow passageway toward the uterus.

The ovaries are also part of the endocrine system because they produce female sex hormones such as estrogen and progesterone.

How does the female reproductive system work?

The female reproductive system enables a woman to produce eggs (ova), have sexual intercourse, protect and nourish a fertilized egg until it is fully developed, and give birth.

Sexual reproduction couldn't happen without the sexual organs called the gonads. Most people think of the gonads as the male testicles. But both sexes have gonads: In females the gonads are the ovaries, which make female gametes (eggs). The male gonads make male gametes (sperm).

When a baby girl is born, her ovaries contain hundreds of thousands of eggs, which remain inactive until puberty begins. At puberty, the pituitary gland (in the central part of the brain) starts making hormones that stimulate the ovaries to make female sex hormones, including estrogen. The secretion of these hormones causes a girl to develop into a sexually mature woman.

Toward the end of puberty, girls begin to release eggs as part of a monthly period called the menstrual cycle. About once a month, during ovulation, an ovary sends a tiny egg into one of the fallopian tubes.

Unless the egg is fertilized by a sperm while in the fallopian tube, the egg leaves the body about 2 weeks later through the uterus—this is menstruation. Blood and tissues from the inner lining of the uterus combine to form the menstrual flow, which in most girls lasts from 3 to 5 days.

What is the male reproductive system?

The male has reproductive organs, or genitals, that are both inside and outside the pelvis. The male genitals include the testicles, the duct system, which is made up of the epididymis and the vas deferens, the accessory glands, which include the seminal vesicles and prostate gland, and the penis.

In a guy who has reached sexual maturity, the two oval-shaped testicles, or testes make and store millions of tiny sperm cells.

The testicles are also part of the endocrine system because they make hormones, including testosterone. Testosterone is a major part of puberty in guys. As a guy makes his way through puberty, his testicles produce more and more of it. Testosterone is the hormone that causes boys to develop deeper voices, bigger muscles, and body and facial hair. It also stimulates the production of sperm.

Alongside the testicles are the epididymis and the vas deferens, which transport sperm. The epididymis and the testicles hang in a pouch-like structure outside the pelvis called the scrotum. This bag of skin helps to regulate the temperature of testicles, which need to be kept cooler than body temperature to produce sperm. The scrotum changes size to maintain the right temperature. When the body is cold, the scrotum shrinks and becomes tighter to hold in body heat. When it's warm, it gets larger and floppier to get rid of extra heat. This happens without a guy ever having to think about it. The brain and the nervous system give the scrotum the cue to change size.

The accessory glands, including the seminal vesicles and the prostate gland, provide fluids that lubricate the duct system and nourish the sperm. The urethra is the channel that carries the sperm (in fluid called semen) to the outside of the body through the penis. The urethra is also part of the urinary system because it is also the channel through which pee passes as it leaves the bladder and exits the body.

The penis is actually made up of two parts: the shaft and the glans. The shaft is the main part of the penis and the glans is the tip (sometimes called the head). At the end of the glans is a small slit or opening, which is where semen and pee exit the body through the urethra. The inside of the penis is made of a spongy tissue that can expand and contract.

How does the male reproductive system work?

The male reproductive system makes semen, releases semen into the reproductive system of the female during sexual intercourse, and produces sex hormones, which help a boy develop into a sexually mature man during puberty.

When a baby boy is born, he has all the parts of his reproductive system in place, but it isn't until puberty that he is able to reproduce. When puberty begins, usually between the ages of 9 and 15, the pituitary gland—located near the brain—secretes hormones that stimulate the testicles to produce testosterone. The production of testosterone brings about many physical changes.

Although the timing of these changes is different for every guy, the stages of puberty generally follow a set sequence. During the first stage of male puberty, the scrotum and testes grow larger. Next, the penis becomes longer and the seminal vesicles and prostate gland grow. Hair begins to grow in the pubic area and later on the face and underarms. During this time, the voice also deepens. Guys also have a growth spurt during puberty as they reach their adult height and weight.

(1,510 words)

Task 1

Read the passage above and answer the following questions.

(1) What is reproduction?

(2) How many types of sex cells are involved in human reproduction?

(3) What is the female reproductive system?

(4) What functions does the female reproductive system provide?

(5) What causes a girl to develop into a sexually mature woman?

(6) What is the male reproductive system?

(7) Which hormone is responsible for masculine features?

(8) What functions does the male reproductive system provide?

Task 2

Please label Figure 5-1 and Figure 5-2 with the medical terms you've learnt in Theme reading 1.

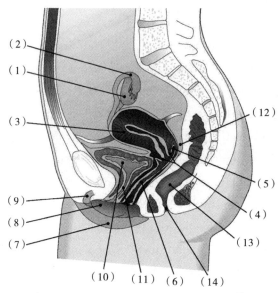

Figure 5-1　Female reproductive system[①]

(1)	(2)
(3)	(4)
(5) posterior fornix	(6)
(7) labium majus	(8) labium minus
(9) clitoris	(10)
(11)	(12) Cul-de-sac
(13) rectum	(14)

① Adapted from *Medical terminology: an illustrated guide (7th edition)*. Cohen, B. J., & DePetris, A. (2014). Philadelphia: Lippincott Williams & Wilkins.

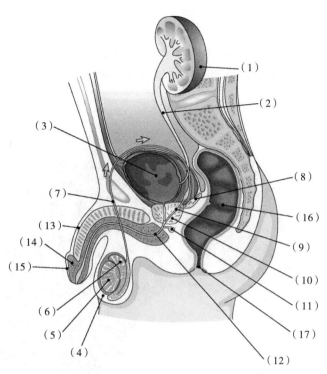

Figure 5-2   Male reproductive system[1]

(1)kidney	(2)ureter
(3)urinary bladder	(4)
(5)	(6)
(7)	(8)
(9)	(10)
(11)bulbourethral (cowper) gland	(12)
(13)	(14)glans penis
(15)prepuce	(16)
(17)anus	

[1]Adapted from *Medical terminology: an illustrated guide (7th edition)*. Cohen, B. J., & DePetris, A. (2014). Philadelphia: Lippincott Williams & Wilkins.

Task 3

Figure 5-3 shows how the fertilization process takes place in humans. Please describe each step by one or two sentences using the numbers as cues and write them down on the blanks below the figure.

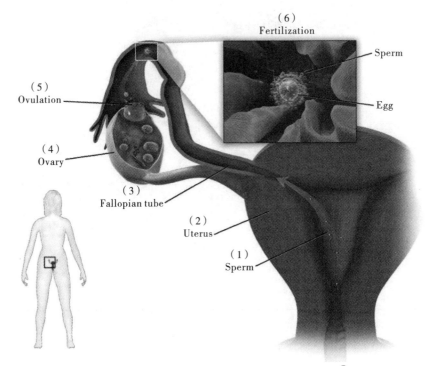

Figure 5-3　Ovulation and fertilization in humans[①]

(1)

(2)

(3)

(4)

(5)

(6)

①Adapted from "Ovulation and fertilization in humans"(n. d.). http://en. volupedia. org

Vocabulary bridge

Study the following terms for common signs, symptoms and diseases related to the reproductive system and translate them into Chinese.

Medical terms	Explanation	Chinese translations
candidiasis	vaginal fungal infection caused by Candida albicans; characterized by a curdy or cheeselike discharge and extreme itching	念珠菌病
cervicitis	inflammation of the uterine cervix	
ectopic pregnancy	implantation of the fertilized ovum outside of the uterine cavity	
endometriosis	presence of endometrial tissue outside (ectopic) the uterine cavity, such as the pelvis or abdomen	
fibroid	benign neoplasm in the uterus that is composed largely of fibrous tissue; also called leiomyoma	
leukorrhea	white discharge from the vagina	
oligomenorrhea	scanty or infrequent menstrual flow	
pregnancy-induced hypertension (PIH)	potentially life-threatening disorder that usually develops after the 20th week of pregnancy and is characterized by edema and proteinuria	
pyosalpinx	pus in the fallopian tube	
retroversion	turning, or state of being turned back, especially an entire organ being tipped from its normal position (such as the uterus)	
sterility	inability of a woman to become pregnant or for a man to impregnate a woman	
toxic shock syndrome (TSS)	rare and sometimes fatal staphylococcus infection that generally occurs in menstruating women, most of whom use vaginal tampons for menstrual protection	
trichomoniasis	protozoal infestation of the vagina, urethra, or prostate	
anorchism	congenital absence of one or both testes; also called anorchia	
balanitis	inflammation of the skin covering the glans penis	
cryptorchidism	failure of one or both testicles to descend into the scrotum	
epispadias	congenital defect in which the urethra opens on upper side of the penis near the glans penis instead of the tip	
hypospadias	congenital defect in which the male urethra opens on undersurface of the penis instead of the tip	
impotence	inability of a man to achieve or maintain a penile erection; commonly called erectile dysfunction	

Medical terms	Explanation	Chinese translations
phimosis	stenosis or narrowness of the preputial orifice so that the foreskin cannot be pushed back over the glans penis	
sexually transmitted disease (STD)	any disease that may be acquired as a result of sexual intercourse or other intimate contact with an infected individual and affects the male and female reproductive systems; also called venereal disease	

Theme reading 2

Ovarian cancer[①]

Cancer is a disease in which abnormal cells in the body grow out of control. Cancer is usually named for the part of the body where it starts, even if it spreads to other body parts later. Ovarian cancer is a group of diseases that originate in the ovaries, or in the related areas of the fallopian tubes and the peritoneum. Women have two ovaries that are located in the pelvis, one on each side of the uterus. The ovaries make female hormones and produce eggs for reproduction. Women have two fallopian tubes that are a pair of long, slender tubes on each side of the uterus. Eggs pass from the ovaries through the fallopian tubes to the uterus. The peritoneum is the tissue lining that covers organs in the abdomen.

Types of ovarian cancer

The ovaries are mainly made up of 3 kinds of cells. Each type of cell can develop into a different type of tumor. Epithelial tumors start from the cells that cover the outer surface of the ovary. Most ovarian tumors are epithelial cell tumors. Germ cell tumors start from the cells that produce the eggs. Stromal tumors start from structural tissue cells that hold the ovary together and produce the female hormones estrogen and progesterone.

Some of these tumors are benign and never spread beyond the ovary. Malignant or borderline ovarian tumors can spread to other parts of the body and can be fatal.

When ovarian cancer is found in its early stages, treatment works best. Ovarian cancer often causes signs and symptoms, so it is important to pay attention to your body and know what is normal for you. Symptoms may be caused by something other than cancer, but the only way to know is to see your doctor, nurse, or other health care professional.

Risk factors

Some mutations can raise your risk for ovarian cancer. Mutations in the breast cancer susceptibility genes 1 and 2 (BRCA1 and BRCA2), and those associated with Lynch syndrome, raise ovarian cancer risk.

---

① Adapted from "Basic Information about Ovarian Cancer"(n.d.). https://www.cdc.gov

There is no way to know for sure if you will get ovarian cancer. Most women get it without being at high risk. However, several factors may increase a woman's risk for ovarian cancer if you are middle-aged or older, or if you have close family members (such as your mother, sister, aunt, or grandmother) on either your mother's or your father's side, who have had ovarian cancer, or if you have a genetic mutation (abnormality) called BRCA1 or BRCA2, or one associated with Lynch syndrome. The risk for ovarian cancer may also increase if you have had breast, uterine, or colorectal cancer, or if you have an Eastern European or Ashkenazi Jewish background, or have endometriosis (a condition where tissue from the lining of the uterus grows elsewhere in the body), or have never given birth or have had trouble getting pregnant.

In addition, some studies suggest that women who take estrogen by itself (without progesterone) for 10 or more years may have an increased risk of ovarian cancer.

If one or more of these factors is true for you, it does not mean you will get ovarian cancer. But you should speak with your doctor about your risk. If you or your family have a history of ovarian cancer, also speak to your doctor about genetic counseling.

Prevention

There is no known way to prevent ovarian cancer, but these things are associated with a lower chance of getting ovarian cancer if you have used birth control pills for five or more years, or have had a tubal ligation (getting your tubes tied), both ovaries removed, or a hysterectomy (an operation in which the uterus, and sometimes the cervix, is removed). There is also a lower chance of getting ovarian cancer if you have given birth or breastfed. Some studies suggest that women who breastfeed for a year or more may have a modestly reduced risk of ovarian cancer.

Talk to your doctor about ways to reduce your risk. While these things may help reduce the chance of getting ovarian cancer, they are not recommended for everybody, and risks and benefits are associated with each. For instance, birth control pills can increase your chance of getting breast cancer. Although you may be able to lower your risk, it does not mean you will not get cancer.

Signs and symptoms

Ovarian cancer may cause the following signs and symptoms. These are vaginal bleeding (particularly if you are past menopause), or discharge from your vagina that is not normal for you, pain or pressure in the pelvic area, abdominal or back pain, bloating, feeling full too quickly, or difficulty eating, a change in your bathroom habits, such as more frequent or urgent need to urinate and/or constipation.

Pay attention to your body, and know what is normal for you. If you have unusual vaginal bleeding, see a doctor right away. If you have any of the other signs for two weeks or longer and they are not normal for you, see a doctor. They may be caused by something other than cancer, but the only way to know is to see a doctor.

Cancer screening

There is no simple and reliable way to screen for ovarian cancer in women who do not have any signs or symptoms.

Screening is when a test is used to look for a disease before there are any symptoms. Cancer screening tests work when they can find disease early, when treatment works best. Diagnostic tests are used when a person has symptoms. The purpose of diagnostic tests is to find out, or diagnose, what is causing the symptoms. Diagnostic tests also may be used to check a person who is considered at high risk for cancer.

The Pap test does not check for ovarian cancer. The only cancer the Pap test screens for is cervical cancer. Since there is no simple and reliable way to screen for any gynecologic cancer except for cervical cancer, it is especially important to recognize warning signs, and learn what you can do to reduce your risk.

Here is what you can do. Pay attention to your body, and know what is normal for you. If you notice any changes in your body that are not normal for you and could be a sign of ovarian cancer, talk to your doctor about them. Ask your doctor if you should have a diagnostic test, like a rectovaginal pelvic exam, a transvaginal ultrasound, or a CA-125 blood test if you have any unexplained signs or symptoms of ovarian cancer. These tests sometimes help find or rule out ovarian cancer.

Treatment

If your doctor says that you have ovarian, fallopian tube, or primary peritoneal cancers, ask to be referred to a gynecologic oncologist—a doctor who was trained to treat cancers of a woman's reproductive system. Gynecologic oncologists can perform surgery on and give chemotherapy (medicine) to women with ovarian cancer. Your doctor can work with you to create a treatment plan.

Treatment for ovarian cancer usually involves a combination of surgery and chemotherapy. Doctors remove cancer tissue in an operation. Special medicines are used to shrink or kill the cancer. The drugs can be pills you take or medicines given in your veins, or sometimes both.

Different treatments may be provided by different doctors on your medical team. Gynecologic oncologists are doctors who have been trained to treat cancers of a woman's reproductive system. They perform surgery and give chemotherapy (medicine). Surgeons are doctors who perform operations. Medical oncologists are doctors who treat cancer with medicine (chemotherapy).

(1,261 words)

Task 1

Read the passage above and answer the following questions.

(1) What is ovarian cancer?

(2) What functions do the ovaries have?

(3) How many types of ovarian tumor are there?

(4) Which tumor type can be fatal?

(5) When does treatment work best?

(6) What are the risk factors for ovarian cancer?

(7) What can be done to reduce the risk of ovarian cancer?

(8) What are the signs and symptoms of ovarian cancer?

(9) What is screening?

(10) What is the purpose of diagnostic tests?

(11) How is ovarian cancer treated?

Task 2

Read the following paragraph carefully and fill in the blanks with the words from the box.

cycles	targeted	vary	shrink	operation
after	stage	scan	damage	treatment

Chemotherapy is the treatment of cancer with anti-cancer drugs. The aim is to destroy cancer cells while causing the least possible (1)_____ to normal, healthy cells. When you have chemotherapy depends on the (2)_____ of the cancer. It may be used at different times. For stage 3 or 4 ovarian cancer, chemotherapy is sometimes given before surgery. This is known as neoadjuvant chemotherapy. The aim is to (3)_____ the tumors to make them easier to remove. After three cycles of chemotherapy, you will have a CT (4)_____ to check how the tumor has responded to the chemotherapy. Your doctor will then decide about having an operation. If you have surgery, you will have another three (5)_____ of chemotherapy afterward. If you do not have surgery, you will continue with a further three cycles of chemotherapy. Chemotherapy is usually given 2 – 4 weeks (6)_____ the surgery (adjuvant chemotherapy) as there may be some cancer cells still in the body. For ovarian cancer, the drugs are usually given in repeating cycles spread over 4 – 5 months, but this can (7)_____ depending on the stage of the cancer and your general health. Your (8)_____ team will talk to you about your specific schedule. Some people may have chemotherapy with a (9)_____ therapy drug. Chemotherapy may be recommended as the main treatment if you are not well enough for a major (10)_____ or when the cancer cannot be surgically removed.

Task 3

Study the boldfaced words in each of the following sentences and make a sentence of your own.

(1) Birth control pills can **increase** your **chance of** getting breast cancer.

Your sentence: <u>Some studies suggest that women who take estrogen by itself (without progesterone) for 10 or more years may **increase** their **chance of** getting ovarian cancer.</u>

(2) Ovarian cancer is a group of diseases that **originates in** the ovaries, or in the related areas of the fallopian tubes and the peritoneum.

Your sentence: _____

_____

(3) Women have two ovaries that **are located in** the pelvis, one on each side of the uterus.

Your sentence: _____

_____

(4) If you notice any changes in your body that are not normal for you and **could be a sign of** ovarian cancer, talk to your doctor about them.

Your sentence: _____

_____

(5) If your doctor says that you have ovarian, fallopian tube, or primary peritoneal cancers, ask to be **referred to** a gynecologic oncologist.

Your sentence: _____

_____

(6) Treatment for ovarian cancer usually **involves a combination of** surgery and chemotherapy.

Your sentence: _____

_____

Task 4

Reorder the following sentences into a reasonable paragraph.

(1) They may include treatments like chemotherapy, hormone therapy, and/or Chinese herbal medicine.

(2) However, a growing number of clinical studies showed Chinese herbal medicine could alleviate chemotherapy-related side effects and improve human immunity.

(3) Chemotherapy kills both tumor and normal cells, leading to many adverse effects.

(4) Adjuvant treatments are necessary to minimize recurrence of ovarian cancer.

(5) Thus it can be a supporting therapy of the adjuvant treatment for ovarian cancer.

Correct order: ____ ____ ____ ____ ____

Story sharing

The following passage① is a plot summary of Margaret Edson's play *Wit*, which follows Vivian Bearing, a renowned professor of seventeenth-century poetry, through her treatment for and final days of advanced metastatic ovarian cancer. Please read the summary and finish the tasks.

Wit—sometimes spelled as *W;t*—is a Pulitzer-Prize winning play by Margaret Edson first published in 1999. The play follows the story of Dr. Vivian Bearing, a fifty-year-old professor of seventeenth-century poetry who has recently been diagnosed with stage-four metastatic ovarian cancer. The plot itself is nonlinear; for example, the opening scene of the play takes place two hours before Vivian dies, but the play switches between Vivian's childhood, career, and treatment milestones to tell her whole story. The final scenes of the play are the only ones that occur in chronological order because Vivian—who has been telling the story to the audience—becomes unconscious as she passes away.

It is worth noting that *Wit* also has an unusual structure that helps shape its themes. Instead of breaking the play into acts, Edson structures her play as one continuous performance. The scenes change around Vivian's monologues, and there is never a break in the action, not even for intermission. Instead, the text of the play is broken up into unnumbered scenes separated by a section break. Additionally, Edson has Vivian speak directly to the audience throughout the play. This technique is called breaking the fourth wall, and Edson uses it to create a connection between Vivian and the audience. Vivian shares her thoughts, feelings, and experiences with the audience to help the audience walk in her shoes.

The plot follows Vivian's life from her diagnosis to her final moments in the hospital. Despite being healthy her whole life, Vivian has recently begun experiencing a combination of exhaustion and abdominal cramps. She decides to go to her gynecologist for a check-up, who suspects Vivian has a tumor. Vivian is referred to Dr. Harvey Kelekian, the chief of medical oncology at her university's hospital. He tells Vivian that she has an aggressive form of cancer and that her best hope of survival comes from an experimental, eight-month treatment. He warns her that the side effects will be severe, but Vivian tells him that he "needn't worry" about her being able to handle it. She decides that at the very least, agreeing to the treatment will help make a "significant contribution" to cancer research.

As Vivian begins her treatment, she takes the audience back to a pivotal encounter she

---

① Adapted from "*Wit* Summary and Study Guide" (n.d.). https://supersummary-production.netlify.app

had with her college professor, Dr. E. M. Ashford. Ashford pushes Vivian to think more critically about Donne's poetry, but she also encourages Vivian to live outside of her studies. Vivian takes Ashford's advice about the former, but not the latter. She tells the audience that after graduate school, she became one of the foremost scholars of Donne's poetry. She chose Donne to prove herself and to recapture the "magic" of language that she first experienced as a young girl. She goes on to become a hard, exacting professor.

In between flashbacks, Vivian walks the audience through her treatment. Her daily care is overseen by her nurse, Susie Monahan, and a young medical oncology fellow, Dr. Jason Posner. On their first meeting, Jason tells Vivian that he took her course as an undergraduate to prove to himself that he could make an A in one of the hardest courses on campus. Like Vivian, Jason loves a challenge; he craves intellectual rigor, which is why he has decided to pursue a career in cancer research. But what Jason has in intelligence, he lacks in compassion. He does not treat Vivian like a sick and possibly dying person; instead, he is more interested in what he can learn about her cancer. Despite interacting with her regularly, he offers her little in the way of comfort. Jason's main concern is that Vivian completes all eight rounds of her chemotherapy drugs, so he can have a complete data set.

Susie, on the other hand, treats Vivian with kindness and compassion. Even though Vivian prides herself on her toughness, her treatment wears down her immune system. When she lands in the ER, Susie swoops in to take care of her. She gets Vivian settled and fetches Jason, who diagnoses her with a secondary infection. Susie pleads with Jason to consult with Dr. Kelekian; Susie thinks they should lower Vivian's dose next cycle. Jason refuses, and he transfers Vivian into isolation instead. Vivian continues to take her chemotherapy at its full dose, but her condition continues to deteriorate.

Vivian begins to realize that she is dying. She often quotes Donne's poetry to help her come to terms with her situation, since Donne's work wrestles with ideas like death, eternity, and salvation. But poetry alone is not enough. Vivian begins reaching out to those around her for comfort. Jason brushes Vivian and her concerns off, but Susie responds with compassion and kindness. Vivian tells Susie she is scared, so Susie helps Vivian make important decisions about her end of life care. Susie asks Vivian what she would like to have happened when her heart stops, and Vivian chooses a "Do Not Resuscitate" order—also known as a DNR. Soon thereafter, Vivian's pain becomes too much to bear, and Dr. Kelekian puts her on a morphine drip.

Vivian receives one last visitor in the hospital: Dr. Ashford, her old mentor. Ashford, now eighty years old, had come to visit Vivian at the university only to find she was in the hospital. Seeing her professor moves Vivian to tears, and Ashford climbs into her hospital bed to comfort her. She holds Vivian as she reads her a children's book, *The Runaway Bunny*, by Margaret Wise Brown. Vivian drifts off to sleep, and Ashford kisses her on the forehead before telling Vivian, "It's time to go. 'And flights of angels sing thee to thy rest'". Then

Ashford leaves.

In the next scene, Jason comes to check on Vivian. He realizes she has no pulse, so he starts CPR and calls in a "Code Blue" to have her resuscitated. Susie rushes in and tries to pull Jason away from Vivian, telling him she has a DNR. Susie tries to call off the code team, but she is too late. As Jason, Susie, and the resuscitation team struggle in the background, Vivian gets out of bed. She unplugs herself from the medical machines and takes off her hat, her medical bracelets, and her dressing gown. She begins walking toward a light shining from offstage. As she reaches for it, the stage lights go dark and the play ends.

(945 words)

Task 1

Read the passage above and write a paragraph to complete it, with the first sentence being provided.

In *Wit*, Vivian is concerned with mortality—both the mortality of her physical body and of her body of scholarly work.

_____

_____

_____

_____

_____

_____

_____

_____

_____

Task 2

Discuss the following questions in groups.

(1) How are Vivian and Jason alike in the play?

(2) How do you think of Dr. Jason Posner's bedside manner?

(3) What is the role of doctors in helping patients make their medical decisions?

(4) What lessons can you learn from Vivian's story?

Vocabulary checklist

英文	中文
* **reproductive** system [ˌriːprəˈdʌktɪv]	生殖系统
organism [ˈɔːgənɪzəm]	有机体，生物
gamete [ˈgæmiːt]	配子
* sperm [spɜːm]	精子
* egg [eg]	卵
* ovum [ˈəʊvəm]	卵
* zygote [ˈzaɪgəʊt]	受精卵
* embryo [ˈembriəʊ]	胚胎
* fetus [ˈfiːtəs]	胎儿
vulva [ˈvʌlvə]	外阴
* vagina [vəˈdʒaɪnə]	阴道
mons pubis [ˌmɒnz ˈpjuːbɪs]	阴阜
labia [ˈleɪbɪə]	阴唇
clitoris [ˈklɪtərɪs]	阴蒂
* sensory [ˈsensəri]	感觉的

英文	中文
* urethra [juˈriːθrə]	尿道
* bladder [ˈblædə(r)]	膀胱
* uterus [ˈjuːtərəs]	子宫
* **fallopian** tube [fəˈləʊpiən]	输卵管
* ovary [ˈəʊvəri]	卵巢
* muscular [ˈmʌskjələ(r)]	肌肉的
mucous membrane [ˈmjuːkəs ˈmembreɪn]	黏膜
* womb [wuːm]	子宫
* cervix [ˈsɜːvɪks]	子宫颈
ovulation [ˌɒvjuˈleɪʃn]	排卵
* **endocrine** system [ˈendəʊkrɪn]	内分泌系统
* hormone [ˈhɔːməʊn]	激素
* estrogen [ˈiːstrədʒən]	雌激素
progesterone [prəˈdʒestərəʊn]	孕酮
* gonad [ˈgəʊnæd]	性腺
* testicle [ˈtestɪkl]	睾丸

英文	中文
* pituitary gland [pɪˈtjuːɪtəri glænd]	垂体
menstrual cycle [ˈmenstruəl]	月经周期
menstruation [ˌmenstruˈeɪʃn]	月经
genitals [ˈdʒenɪtlz]	生殖器
duct [dʌkt]	导管
epididymis [ˌepɪˈdɪdɪmɪs]	附睾
vas deferens [ˌvæs ˈdefərenz]	输精管
seminal vesicle [ˈsemɪnlˈvesɪkl]	精囊
* **prostate** gland [ˈprɒsteɪt]	前列腺
* penis [ˈpiːnɪs]	阴茎
testosterone [teˈstɒstərəʊn]	睾酮
* scrotum [ˈskrəʊtəm]	阴囊
semen [ˈsiːmən]	精液
shaft [ʃɑːft]	阴茎体
glans [glænz]	阴茎头
ovarian cancer [əʊˈveəriən]	卵巢癌

英文	中文
peritoneum [ˌperɪtəˈniːəm]	腹膜
* pelvis [ˌpelvɪs]	骨盆
* abdomen [ˌæbdəmən]	腹部
epithelial tumor [ˌepɪˈθiːlɪəl]	上皮性肿瘤
germ cell tumor [dʒɜːm]	生殖细胞肿瘤
stromal tumor [ˈstrəʊməl]	基质瘤
malignant ovarian tumor [məˈlɪgnənt]	恶性卵巢肿瘤
borderline ovarian tumor [ˈbɔːdəlaɪn]	边缘性卵巢肿瘤
mutation [mjuːˈteɪʃn]	突变
susceptibility [səˌseptəˈbɪləti]	易感性
Lynch syndrome [lɪntʃ ˈsɪndrəʊm]	林奇综合征
uterine cancer [ˈjuːtəraɪn]	子宫癌
colorectal cancer [ˌkəʊləˈrektəl]	结直肠癌
endometriosis [ˌendəʊˌmiːtrɪˈəʊsɪs]	子宫内膜异位
tubal **ligation** [laɪˈgeɪʃn]	输卵管结扎
hysterectomy [ˌhɪstəˈrektəmi]	子宫切除术
menopause [ˈmenəpɔːz]	绝经期

英文	中文
bloating [ˈbləʊtɪŋ]	胃气胀
＊constipation [ˌkɒnstɪˈpeɪʃn]	便秘
Pap test [pæp]	宫颈刮片检查,巴氏涂片检查
cervical cancer [ˈsɜːvɪkl]	子宫颈癌
gynecologic cancer [ˌgaɪnəkəˈlɒdʒɪk]	妇科癌症
rectovaginal pelvic exam [ˈrektəʊvæˈdʒaɪnl]	直肠阴道盆腔检查
transvaginal ultrasound [ˌtrænsvəˈdʒaɪnəl]	经阴道超声
primary **peritoneal** cancer [ˌperɪtəʊˈniːəl]	原发性腹膜癌
gynecologic oncologist [ˌgaɪnəkəˈlɒdʒɪk ɒŋˈkɒlədʒɪst]	妇科肿瘤学家
＊chemotherapy [ˌkiːməʊˈθerəpi]	化学疗法
＊vein [veɪn]	静脉
metastatic ovarian cancer [ˌmetəˈstætɪk]	转移性卵巢癌
abdominal **cramp** [kræmp]	痉挛性腹痛
oncology [ɒŋˈkɒlədʒi]	肿瘤学
＊**immune** system [ɪˈmjuːn]	免疫系统
secondary **infection** [ɪnˈfekʃn]	继发感染
morphine [ˈmɔːfiːn]	吗啡

注：＊表示高频医学英语词汇。

Chapter 6

Endocrine system

Learning objectives

Upon completion of this chapter, you will be able to

❖ name major endocrine organs and tell their functions;

❖ describe the functions of the endocrine system;

❖ list major conditions affecting the endocrine system;

❖ understand information about diabetes;

❖ gather information about common endocrine diseases;

❖ present one common endocrine disease with group members.

Theme reading 1

An introduction to the endocrine system[1]

What is the endocrine system?

The endocrine system is made up of glands that make hormones. Hormones are the body's chemical messengers. They carry information and instructions from one set of cells to another.

Hormones are produced in extremely small amounts and are highly potent. By means of their actions on various target tissues, they affect growth, metabolism, reproductive activity, and behavior.

Chemically, hormones fall into two categories: steroid hormones, which are made from lipids and amino acid hormones, which include proteins and protein-like compounds. Steroids are produced by the sex glands (gonads) and the outer region (cortex) of the adrenal glands. All of the endocrine glands aside from the gonads and adrenal cortex produce amino acid

---

① Adapted from "Endocrine System." Hirsch, L. (2018). https://kidshealth.org

hormones. The production of hormones is controlled mainly by negative feedback—that is, the hormone itself, or some product of hormone activity, acts as a control over further manufacture of the hormone—a self-regulating system. Hormone production may also be controlled by the nervous system or by other hormones.

What does the endocrine system do?

The endocrine system influences almost every cell, organ, and function of our bodies. Endocrine glands release hormones into the bloodstream. This lets the hormones travel to cells in other parts of the body. The endocrine hormones help control mood, growth and development, the way our organs work, metabolism, and reproduction.

The endocrine system regulates how much of each hormone is released. This can depend on levels of hormones already in the blood, or on levels of other substances in the blood, like calcium. Many things affect hormone levels, such as stress, infection, and changes in the balance of fluid and minerals in blood.

Too much or too little of any hormone can harm the body. Medicines can treat many of these problems.

What are the major parts of the endocrine system?

While many parts of the body make hormones, the major glands that make up the endocrine system are

- hypothalamus;
- pituitary;
- thyroid;
- parathyroids;
- adrenals;
- pineal;
- ovaries;
- testes (the plural of testis);
- pancreas.

Hypothalamus

The hypothalamus is in the lower central part of the brain. It links the endocrine system and nervous system. Nerve cells in the hypothalamus make chemicals that control the release of hormones secreted from the pituitary gland. The hypothalamus gathers information sensed by the brain (such as the surrounding temperature, light exposure, and feelings) and sends it to the pituitary. This information influences the hormones that the pituitary makes and releases.

Pituitary

The pituitary gland is at the base of the brain, and is no bigger than a pea. Despite its small size, the pituitary is often called the "master gland." The hormones it makes control many other endocrine glands. The pituitary gland secretes many hormones, such as

- growth hormone, which stimulates the growth of bone and other body tissues and plays a role in the body's handling of nutrients and minerals;
- prolactin, which activates milk production in women who are breastfeeding;
- thyrotropin, which stimulates the thyroid gland to make thyroid hormones;
- corticotropin, which stimulates the adrenal gland to make certain hormones;
- antidiuretic hormone, which helps control body water balance through its effect on the kidneys;
- oxytocin, which triggers the contractions of the uterus that happen during labor.

The pituitary also secretes endorphins, chemicals that act on the nervous system and reduce feelings of pain. The pituitary also secretes hormones that signal the reproductive organs to make sex hormones. The pituitary gland also controls ovulation and the menstrual cycle in women.

Thyroid

The thyroid is in the front part of the lower neck. It's shaped like a bow tie or butterfly. It makes the thyroid hormones thyroxine and triiodothyronine. These hormones control the rate at which cells burn fuels from food to make energy. The more thyroid hormone there is in the bloodstream, the faster chemical reactions happen in the body.

Hyperthyroidism (overactive thyroid) occurs when your thyroid gland produces too much of the hormone thyroxine. Hyperthyroidism can accelerate your body's metabolism, causing unintentional weight loss and a rapid or irregular heartbeat.

Hypothyroidism (underactive thyroid) is a condition in which your thyroid gland doesn't produce enough of certain crucial hormones. Hypothyroidism may not cause noticeable symptoms in the early stages. Over time, untreated hypothyroidism can cause a number of health problems, such as obesity, joint pain, infertility and heart disease.

Parathyroids

Attached to the thyroid are four tiny glands that work together called the parathyroids. They release parathyroid hormone, which controls the level of calcium in the blood with the help of calcitonin, which the thyroid makes.

Adrenal glands

These two triangular adrenal glands sit on top of each kidney. The adrenal glands have two parts, each of which makes a set of hormones and has a different function.

The outer part is the adrenal cortex. It makes hormones called corticosteroids that help control salt and water balance in the body, the body's response to stress, metabolism, the immune system, and sexual development and function.

The inner part is the adrenal medulla. It makes catecholamines, such as epinephrine. Also called adrenaline, epinephrine increases blood pressure and heart rate when the body is under stress.

Pineal

The pineal body, also called the pineal gland, is in the middle of the brain. It secretes melatonin, a hormone that may help regulate when you sleep at night and when you wake in the morning.

Reproductive glands

Reproductive glands are the main source of sex hormones. Most people don't realize it, but both guys and girls have gonads. In guys the male gonads, or testes, are in the scrotum. They secrete hormones called androgens, the most important of which is testosterone. These hormones tell a guy's body when it's time to make the changes associated with puberty, like penis and height growth, deepening voice, and growth in facial and pubic hair. Working with hormones from the pituitary gland, testosterone also tells a guy's body when it's time to make sperm in the testes.

A girl's gonads, the ovaries, are in her pelvis. They make eggs and secrete the female hormones estrogen and progesterone. Estrogen is involved when a girl starts puberty. During puberty, a girl will have breast growth, start to accumulate body fat around the hips and thighs, and have a growth spurt. Estrogen and progesterone are also involved in the regulation of a girl's menstrual cycle. These hormones also play a role in pregnancy.

Pancreas

The pancreas makes insulin and glucagon, which are hormones that control the level of glucose, or sugar, in the blood. Insulin helps keep the body supplied with stores of energy. The body uses this stored energy for exercise and activity, and it also helps organs work as they should.

How can I keep my endocrine system healthy?

Here are some ways to help keep your endocrine system healthy:

• Get plenty of exercise.

• Eat a nutritious diet.

• Go for regular medical checkups.

• Talk to the doctor before taking any supplements or herbal treatments.

• Let the doctor know about any family history of endocrine problems, such as diabetes or thyroid problems.

(1,167 words)

Task 1

Read the passage above and answer the following questions.

(1) What is the endocrine system?

(2) What can hormones do?

(3) What does the endocrine system do?

(4)What are the major parts of the endocrine system?

(5)Which part of the endocrine system is the "master gland"?

(6)What can you do to keep your endocrine system healthy?

Task 2

Please label Figure 6-1 with the medical terms you've learnt in Theme reading 1.

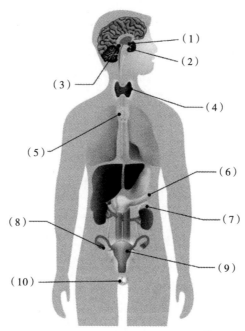

(1)

(2)

(3)

(4)

(5)

(6)

(7)

(8)

(9)

(10)

Figure 6-1   The endocrine system[①]

(1)	(2)
(3)	(4)
(5)	(6)
(7)	(8)
(9)	(10)

---

①Adapted from "The endocrine system"(n.d.). https://www.epa.gov

Task 3

Please fill in the following table with the information in Theme reading 1.

Glands	Location	Hormones	Primary functions
Hypothalamus	in the lower central part of the brain	antidiuretic hormone	helps control body water balance through its effect on the kidneys
Pituitary gland			
Thyroid			
Parathyroids			
Adrenal glands			
Pineal gland			
Ovaries			
Testes			
Pancreas	behind the stomach		

Vocabulary bridge

Study the following terms for common signs, symptoms and diseases related to the endocrine system and translate them into Chinese.

Medical terms	Explanation	Chinese translations
Addison disease	relatively uncommon chronic disorder caused by deficiency of cortical hormones that results when the adrenal cortex is damaged or atrophied	艾迪生病
Cushing syndrome	cluster of symptoms caused by excessive amounts of cortisol or adrenocorticotropic hormone (ACTH) circulating in the blood	

Medical terms	Explanation	Chinese translations
diabetes mellitus (DM)	chronic metabolic disorder of impaired carbohydrate, protein, and fat metabolism due to insufficient production of insulin or the body's inability to utilize insulin properly	
exophthalmos	abnormal protrusion of the eyeball(s), possibly due to thyrotoxicosis, tumor of the orbit, orbital cellulitis, leukemia, or aneurysm	
Graves disease	multisystem autoimmune disorder that involves growth of the thyroid (hyperthyroidism) associated with hypersecretion of thyroxine; also called exophthalmic goiter, thyrotoxicosis, or toxic goiter	
myxedema	advanced hypothyroidism in adults that results from hypofunction of the thyroid gland and affects body fluids, causing edema and increasing blood volume and blood pressure	
obesity	excessive accumulation of fat that exceeds the body's skeletal and physical standards, usually an increase of 20% or more above ideal body weight	
pituitarism	any disorder of the pituitary gland and its function	

Theme reading 2

Diabetes[①]

What is diabetes?

Diabetes is a chronic (long-lasting) health condition that affects how your body turns food into energy.

Your body breaks down most of the food you eat into sugar (glucose) and releases it into your bloodstream. When your blood sugar goes up, it signals your pancreas to release insulin. Insulin acts like a key to let the blood sugar into your body's cells for use as energy.

With diabetes, your body doesn't make enough insulin or can't use it as well as it should. When there isn't enough insulin or cells stop responding to insulin, too much blood sugar stays in your bloodstream. Over time, that can cause serious health problems, such as heart disease, vision loss, and kidney disease.

Types of diabetes

There are three main types of diabetes: type 1, type 2, and gestational diabetes (diabetes while pregnant).

---

①Adapted from "What is diabetes?" (n. d.). https://www.cdc.gov

Type 1 diabetes

Type 1 diabetes is thought to be caused by an autoimmune reaction (the body attacks itself by mistake) that stops your body from making insulin. Approximately 5%–10% of the people who have diabetes have type 1. Symptoms of type 1 diabetes often develop quickly. It's usually diagnosed in children, teens, and young adults. If you have type 1 diabetes, you'll need to take insulin every day to survive. Currently, no one knows how to prevent type 1 diabetes.

Type 2 diabetes

With type 2 diabetes, your body doesn't use insulin well and can't keep blood sugar at normal levels. About 90%–95% of people with diabetes have type 2. It develops over many years and is usually diagnosed in adults (but more and more in children, teens, and young adults). You may not notice any symptoms, so it's important to get your blood sugar tested if you're at risk. Type 2 diabetes can be prevented or delayed with healthy lifestyle changes, such as losing weight, eating healthy food, and being active.

Gestational diabetes

Gestational diabetes develops in pregnant women who have never had diabetes. If you have gestational diabetes, your baby could be at higher risk for health problems. Gestational diabetes usually goes away after your baby is born but increases your risk for type 2 diabetes later in life. Your baby is more likely to have obesity as a child or teen, and more likely to develop type 2 diabetes later in life too.

Prediabetes

In the United States, 88 million adults—more than 1 in 3—have prediabetes. What's more, more than 84% of them don't know they have it. With prediabetes, blood sugar levels are higher than normal, but not high enough yet to be diagnosed as type 2 diabetes. Prediabetes raises your risk for type 2 diabetes, heart disease, and stroke. The good news is if you have prediabetes, a CDC-recognized lifestyle change program can help you take healthy steps to reverse it.

Diabetes symptoms

If you have any of the following diabetes symptoms, see your doctor about getting your blood sugar tested:

- urinating (peeing) a lot, often at night
- being very thirsty
- losing weight without trying
- being very hungry
- having blurry vision
- having numb or tingling hands or feet
- feeling very tired
- having very dry skin

- having sores that heal slowly
- having more infections than usual

Risk factors

Risk factors for type 1 diabetes

Although the exact cause of type 1 diabetes is unknown, factors that may signal an increased risk include:

- Family history. Your risk increases if a parent or sibling has type 1 diabetes.
- Geography. Certain countries, such as Finland and Sweden, have higher rates of type 1 diabetes.

Risk factors for prediabetes and type 2 diabetes

Researchers don't fully understand why some people develop prediabetes and type 2 diabetes and others don't. It's clear that certain factors increase the risk, however, including:

- Weight. The fattier tissue you have, the more resistant your cells become to insulin.
- Inactivity. The less active you are, the greater your risk. Physical activity helps you control your weight, uses up glucose as energy and makes your cells more sensitive to insulin.
- Family history. Your risk increases if a parent or sibling has type 2 diabetes.
- Race or ethnicity. Although it's unclear why, certain people—including Black, Hispanic, American Indian and Asian American people—are at higher risk.
- Age. Your risk increases as you get older. This may be because you tend to exercise less, lose muscle mass and gain weight as you age. But type 2 diabetes is also increasing among children, adolescents and younger adults.

Complications

Long-term complications of diabetes develop gradually. The longer you have diabetes and the less controlled your blood sugar—the higher the risk of complications. Eventually, diabetes complications may be disabling or even life-threatening. Possible complications include:

- Cardiovascular disease. Diabetes dramatically increases the risk of various cardiovascular problems, including coronary artery disease with chest pain (angina), heart attack, stroke and narrowing of arteries (atherosclerosis). If you have diabetes, you're more likely to have heart disease or stroke.
- Nerve damage (neuropathy). Excess sugar can injure the walls of the tiny blood vessels (capillaries) that nourish your nerves, especially in your legs. This can cause tingling, numbness, burning or pain that usually begins at the tips of the toes or fingers and gradually spreads upward. Left untreated, you could lose all sense of feeling in the affected limbs. Damage to the nerves related to digestion can cause problems with nausea, vomiting, diarrhea or constipation. For men, it may lead to erectile dysfunction.
- Kidney damage (nephropathy). The kidneys contain millions of tiny blood vessel

clusters (glomeruli) that filter waste from your blood. Diabetes can damage this delicate filtering system. Severe damage can lead to kidney failure or irreversible end-stage kidney disease, which may require dialysis or a kidney transplant.

• Eye damage (retinopathy). Diabetes can damage the blood vessels of the retina (diabetic retinopathy), potentially leading to blindness. Diabetes also increases the risk of other serious vision conditions, such as cataracts and glaucoma.

• Foot damage. Nerve damage in the feet or poor blood flow to the feet increases the risk of various foot complications. Left untreated, cuts and blisters can develop serious infections, which often heal poorly. These infections may ultimately require toe, foot or leg amputation.

• Skin conditions. Diabetes may leave you more susceptible to skin problems, including bacterial and fungal infections.

• Hearing impairment. Hearing problems are more common in people with diabetes.

• Alzheimer's disease. Type 2 diabetes may increase the risk of dementia, such as Alzheimer's disease. The poorer your blood sugar control, the greater the risk appears to be. Although there are theories as to how these disorders might be connected, none has yet been proved.

• Depression. Depression symptoms are common in people with type 1 and type 2 diabetes. Depression can affect diabetes management.

Prevention

Type 1 diabetes can't be prevented. However, the same healthy lifestyle choices that help treat prediabetes, type 2 diabetes and gestational diabetes can also help prevent them:

• Eat healthy foods. Choose foods lower in fat and calories and higher in fiber. Focus on fruits, vegetables and whole grains. Strive for variety to prevent boredom.

• Get more physical activity. Aim for about 30 minutes of moderate aerobic activity on most days of the week, or at least 150 minutes of moderate aerobic activity a week.

• Lose excess pounds. If you're overweight, losing even 7% of your body weight, for example, 14 pounds (6.4 kilograms) if you weigh 200 pounds (90.7 kilograms), can reduce the risk of diabetes. Don't try to lose weight during pregnancy, however. Talk to your doctor about how much weight is healthy for you to gain during pregnancy. To keep your weight in a healthy range, focus on permanent changes to your eating and exercise habits. Motivate yourself by remembering the benefits of losing weight, such as a healthier heart, more energy and improved self-esteem.

• Sometimes medication is an option as well. Oral diabetes drugs such as metformin may reduce the risk of type 2 diabetes, but healthy lifestyle choices remain essential. Have your blood sugar checked at least once a year to check that you haven't developed type 2 diabetes.

(1,342 words)

Task 1

Read the passage above and answer the following questions.

(1) What is diabetes?

(2) What causes diabetes?

(3) How does insulin work?

(4) What are the main different types of diabetes?

(5) What are the symptoms of diabetes?

(6) What are the risk factors for type 2 diabetes?

(7) What are the possible complications of diabetes?

(8) Can type 1 diabetes be prevented?

(9) How can type 2 diabetes be prevented?

Task 2

Read the following paragraph carefully and fill in the blanks with the words from the box.

immune system	monitor	hyperglycemia	make	use
gestational diabetes	types	heart disease	blood	insulin

Diabetes is a disease in which your blood glucose, or blood sugar, levels are too high. Glucose comes from the food you eat. (1)_____ is a hormone that helps the glucose get into your cells to give them energy. The main cause of diabetes varies by (2)_____ . The most common types of diabetes are type 1 and type 2 diabetes. With type 1 diabetes, your body does not (3)_____ insulin. Your (4)_____ attacks and destroys the cells in your pancreas that make insulin. With type 2 diabetes, the more common type, your body does not (5)_____ insulin properly. Without enough insulin, the glucose stays in your (6)_____ . Over time, having too much glucose in your blood can cause serious problems. (7)_____ , also called raised blood glucose or raised blood sugar, is a common effect of uncontrolled diabetes. Diabetes can also cause (8)_____ , stroke and even the need to remove a limb. Pregnant women can also get diabetes, called (9)_____ . Blood tests can show if you have diabetes. One type of test, the A1C, can also check on how you are managing your diabetes. Exercise, weight control and sticking to your meal plan can help control your diabetes. You should also (10)_____ your blood glucose level and take medicine if prescribed.

Task 3

Study the boldfaced words in each of the following sentences and make a sentence of your own.

(1) Most of the food you eat is **broken down** into sugar (also called glucose) and released into your bloodstream.

Your sentence: <u>Osteoporosis occurs when too much spongy bone tissue (which is found inside of most bones) is **broken down** and not enough new bone material is made.</u>

(2) Diabetes is a chronic (long-lasting) health condition that affects how your body **turns** food **into** energy.

Your sentence: _____

_____

(3) Glucose is a source of energy for the cells that **make up** muscles and other tissues.

Your sentence: _____

_____

(4) When your blood sugar **goes up**, it signals your pancreas to release insulin.

Your sentence: _____

_____

(5) Diabetes also **increases the risk of** other serious vision conditions, such as cataracts and glaucoma.

Your sentence: _____

_____

(6) Having blood pressure over 140/90 millimeters of mercury (mmHg) **is linked to** an increased risk of type 2 diabetes.

Your sentence: _____

_____

Task 4

Reorder the following sentences into a reasonable paragraph.

(1) Controlling blood sugar can keep you and your baby healthy and prevent a difficult delivery.

(2) Like other types of diabetes, gestational diabetes affects how your cells use sugar (glucose).

(3) During pregnancy you can help control gestational diabetes by eating healthy foods, exercising and, if necessary, taking medication.

(4) Gestational diabetes is diabetes diagnosed for the first time during pregnancy

(gestation).

(5) While any pregnancy complication is concerning, there's good news.

(6) Gestational diabetes causes high blood sugar that can affect your pregnancy and your baby's health.

Correct order: ____　____　____　____　____　____

Story sharing

The following passage[①] by James P. Brody, a professor of biomedical engineering at the University of California, Irvine for over 20 years, describes the discovery of insulin by the joint efforts of several scientists. Please read the passage and finish the tasks.

Diabetes was a fatal disease before insulin was discovered in 1921. A century ago, people diagnosed with this metabolic disorder usually survived only a few years. Physicians had no way to treat their diabetic patients' dangerously high blood sugar levels, which were due to a lack of the hormone insulin. Today, though, nearly 1.6 million Americans are living normal lives with Type 1 diabetes thanks to the discovery of insulin.

This medical breakthrough is usually attributed to one person, Frederick Banting, who was searching for a cure for diabetes. But getting a reliable diabetes treatment depended on the research of two other scientists, Oskar Minkowski and Søren Sørensen, who had done earlier research on seemingly unrelated topics.

Basic research pointed to the pancreas

Diabetes had been known since antiquity. The first symptoms were often a prodigious thirst and urination. Within weeks the patient would be losing weight. Within months, the patient would enter a coma, then die. For centuries, no one had any clue about what caused diabetes.

People had, though, been aware of the pancreas for centuries. The Greek anatomist Herophilos first described it around 300 BCE. Based on its anatomical location, people suspected it was involved in the digestive system. But no one knew whether the pancreas was an essential organ, like the stomach, or extraneous, like the appendix.

In 1889, Oskar Minkowski, a pathologist at the University of Strassburg, in what was then Germany, was one of the most talented surgeons of his time. As part of a study, he performed a surgical feat that was thought to be impossible: keeping an animal alive after totally removing its pancreas.

---

① Adapted from "Insulin was discovered 100 years ago." Brody, J. P. (2021). https://www.asbmb.org

The dog he operated on survived the surgery, but to Minkowski's surprise, it began exhibiting all the symptoms of diabetes. Minkowski had discovered that removing the pancreas caused diabetes. Today, this is known as an animal model of the disease. Once an animal model of a disease is established, researchers can experiment with different cures in the animal in hopes they'll find something that will then work in people.

Can you grind up a pancreas and feed it to a diabetic animal to cure or alleviate the symptoms of diabetes? No, that didn't work. The problem, understood in today's terms, is that the pancreas has two functions: producing enzymes for the digestive system and producing insulin. Mixed together, the digestive enzymes destroyed the insulin.

Isolating the insulin

In 1920, Frederick Banting, a small-town doctor in London, Ontario, had an idea. He thought that he could surgically tie off the ducts between the pancreas and the digestive system in an animal. Wait for a few weeks, while the part of the pancreas that produces those digestive enzymes decays, then remove the pancreas completely. This decayed pancreas, he thought, would contain the insulin, but not the destructive enzymes.

On July 27, 1921, he concluded this experiment in the laboratory of J. J. R. Macleod at the University of Toronto. Banting, working with a Toronto student named Charles Best, prepared an extract from the atrophied pancreas of a dog. Then he injected the extract into another dog that had induced diabetes, due to the removal of its pancreas. The animal's diabetes symptoms began to disappear.

Although Banting's experiment was successful, his method of insulin purification was impractical. J. J. R. Macleod assigned the biochemist James Collip the task of coming up with a practical method of purifying insulin from a pancreas.

Collip developed a method based on alcohol purification. The concept was simple: He'd mash up a fresh pig pancreas, readily available from butcher shops, and mix it into a solution of alcohol and water. Collip slowly increased the percentage of alcohol in the solution. He found that the insulin would stay dissolved in the solution until he reached a critical concentration of alcohol, then it would suddenly fall out of solution, no longer dissolved in the liquid. By collecting that solid precipitate at the bottom of a flask, he had a purified form of insulin.

Collip's extraction of insulin allowed Banting and others at the University of Toronto Hospital to begin treating patients. The first injections took place in January 1922. Within weeks, the results were miraculous. These injections of insulin helped dozens of patients who were close to dying regain normal activities. Word spread. Demand for insulin increased.

Insight from a brewery

But disaster struck when Collip failed to purify larger batches of insulin. He was puzzled why, following the exact same recipe as he'd used before, his preparations lacked insulin. J. J. R. Macleod now turned to Eli Lilly and Company, a commercial firm in Indiana that made medicinal capsules, for help.

At Eli Lilly, the purification problem fell to George Walden, a 27-year-old chemist. Walden thought of a measure that Danish chemist Søren Sørensen had introduced a dozen years before.

Sørensen was the director in the early 1900s of the Carlsberg Laboratory, set up by the beer company to advance the science of brewing. He introduced the concept of pH as a way to quantify the acidity of a solution. A higher pH during the brewing stage leads to a more bitter-tasting beer.

When Walden measured the pH of the pancreas solution, he discovered that the acidity was far more important to the solubility of insulin than the alcohol concentration. He set up a purification procedure like Collip's but based on pH rather than alcohol concentration. Collip's failure to scale up purification of insulin was probably because he neglected to control the pH of the solution carefully.

This insight allowed for mass production of insulin.

(1,002 words)

Task 1

Read the passage above and write a paragraph to complete it, with the first sentence being provided.

By May 1924, diabetes was no longer a fatal disease.

_____

_____

_____

_____

_____

_____

_____

_____

_____

_____

_____

Task 2

Discuss the following questions in groups.

(1) How was an animal model of diabetes established by Minkowski?

(2) How was insulin isolated from pancreas?

(3) How was the mass production of insulin made possible?

(4) What can you learn from the story of overcoming diabetes, the implacable enemies of men in the past?

Vocabulary checklist

英文	中文
* **endocrine** system [ˈendəʊkrɪn]	内分泌系统
* gland [glænd]	腺
* reproductive [ˌriːprəˈdʌktɪv]	生殖的
* **steroid** hormone [ˈsterɔɪd ˈhɔːməʊn]	类固醇激素
lipid [ˈlɪpɪd]	脂质
amino acid [əˈmiːnəʊ]	氨基酸
* protein [ˈprəʊtiːn]	蛋白质
* gonad [ˈgəʊnæd]	性腺,生殖腺
cortex [ˈkɔːteks]	皮质
* **adrenal** gland [əˈdriːnl]	肾上腺
adrenal cortex	肾上腺皮质

英文	中文
＊ hypothalamus [ˌhaɪpə'θæləməs]	下丘脑
＊ pituitary [pɪ'tjuːɪtəri]	垂体
＊ thyroid ['θaɪrɔɪd]	甲状腺;甲状腺的
＊ parathyroid [ˌpærə'θaɪrɔɪd]	甲状旁腺
＊ pineal [paɪ'niːəl]	松果体;松果体的
＊ ovary ['əʊvəri]	卵巢
＊ testis ['testɪs]	睾丸
＊ pancreas ['pæŋkriəs]	胰腺
＊ secrete [sɪ'kriːt]	分泌
prolactin [prəʊ'læktɪn]	催乳素
thyrotropin [θaɪ'rɒtrəpɪn]	促甲状腺激素
corticotropin [ˌkɔːtɪkəʊ'trəʊpɪn]	促肾上腺皮质激素
antidiuretic hormone [ˌæntɪˌdaɪjʊə'retɪk]	抗利尿剂激素
oxytocin [ˌɒksɪ'təʊsɪn]	催产素,缩宫素
endorphin [en'dɔːfɪn]	内啡肽
ovulation [ˌɒvju'leɪʃn]	排卵

英文	中文
menstrual cycle [ˈmenstruəl]	月经周期
＊ thyroxine [θaɪˈrɒksiːn]	甲状腺素
triiodothyronine [traɪˌaɪədəʊˈθaɪrəniːn]	三碘甲状腺原氨酸
hyperthyroidism [haɪpəˈθaɪrɔɪdɪzəm]	甲状腺功能亢进
hypothyroidism [haɪpəʊˈθaɪrɔɪdɪzəm]	甲状腺功能减退
calcitonin [ˌkælsɪˈtəʊnɪn]	降钙素
corticosteroid [ˌkɔːtɪkəʊˈstɪərɔɪd]	皮质类固醇
adrenal medulla [əˈdriːnl meˈdʌlə]	肾上腺髓质
catecholamine [ˌkætəˈkɒləˌmiːn]	儿茶酚胺
epinephrine [ˌepɪˈnefrɪn]	肾上腺素
adrenaline [əˈdrenəlɪn]	肾上腺素
＊ melatonin [ˌmeləˈtəʊnɪn]	褪黑素
＊ scrotum [ˈskrəʊtəm]	阴囊
＊ androgen [ˈændrədʒən]	雄激素
testosterone [teˈstɒstərəʊn]	睾酮,睾丸素
＊ puberty [ˈpjuːbəti]	青春期

英文	中文
* penis [ˈpiːnɪs]	阴茎
* pelvis [ˈpelvɪs]	骨盆
* estrogen [ˈiːstrədʒən]	雌激素
progesterone [prəˈdʒestərəʊn]	黄体酮
* insulin [ˈɪnsjəlɪn]	胰岛素
* glucagon [ˈgluːkəgɒn]	胰高血糖素
* glucose [ˈgluːkəʊs]	葡萄糖
* diabetes [daɪəˈbiːtiːz]	糖尿病
gestational diabetes [dʒeˈsteɪʃənəl]	孕期糖尿病
autoimmune reaction [ɔːtəʊɪˈmjuːn]	自身免疫反应
prediabetes [ˌpriːdaɪəˈbiːtiːz]	前驱糖尿病
* urinate [ˈjʊərɪneɪt]	排尿
blurry vision [ˈblɜːri]	视物模糊
numb [nʌm]	麻木的
tingling [ˈtɪŋglɪŋ]	刺痛的
* cardiovascular [ˌkɑːdiəʊˈvæskjələ(r)]	心血管的

英文	中文
* **coronary artery** disease [ˈkɒrənri][ˈɑːtəri]	冠状动脉疾病
angina [ænˈdʒaɪnə]	心绞痛
* heart attack	心脏病发作
* stroke [strəʊk]	脑卒中
* atherosclerosis [ˌæθərəʊskləˈrəʊsɪs]	动脉粥样硬化
neuropathy [njʊˈrɒpəθi]	神经病变
* capillary [kəˈpɪləri]	毛细血管
* diarrhea [daɪəˈrɪə]	腹泻
* constipation [kɒnstɪˈpeɪʃn]	便秘
erectile dysfunction [ɪˈrektaɪl]	勃起功能障碍
nephropathy [neˈfrɒpəθi]	肾病
glomeruli [gləʊˈmerjʊlaɪ]	肾小球（glomerulus 的复数）
retinopathy [ˌretɪˈnɒpəθi]	视网膜病变
retina [ˈretɪnə]	视网膜
cataract [ˈkætərækt]	白内障
glaucoma [glɔːˈkəʊmə]	青光眼
* **Alzheimer's** disease [ˈæltshaɪməz]	阿尔茨海默病

英文	中文
＊dementia [dɪˈmenʃə]	痴呆
metformin [metˈfɔmɪn]	二甲双胍(抗糖尿病药、降血糖药)
＊urination [ˌjʊərɪˈneɪʃn]	排尿
＊anatomist [əˈnætəmɪst]	解剖学家
＊appendix [əˈpendɪks]	阑尾
＊pathologist [pəˈθɒlədʒɪst]	病理学家,病理学医生
＊enzyme [ˈenzaɪm]	酶
＊duct [dʌkt]	导管
decay [dɪˈkeɪ]	腐烂
atrophied [ˈætrəfɪd]	萎缩的
concentration [ˌkɒnsnˈtreɪʃn]	浓度
precipitate [prɪˈsɪpɪteɪt]	沉淀物,析出物
acidity [əˈsɪdəti]	酸度

注:＊表示高频医学英语词汇。

Chapter 7

Nervous system

Upon completion of this chapter, you will be able to

❖ name the parts of the brain;

❖ describe the main structure of the nervous system;

❖ list common diseases related to the nervous system;

❖ understand information about Alzheimer's disease;

❖ gather information about common nervous system diseases;

❖ present one common nervous system disease with group members.

Theme reading 1

An introduction to the nervous system①

What does the brain do?

The brain controls what you think and feel, how you learn and remember, and the way you move and talk. But it also controls things you're less aware of—like the beating of your heart and the digestion of your food.

Think of the brain as a central computer that controls all the body's functions. The rest of the nervous system is like a network that relays messages back and forth from the brain to different parts of the body. It does this via the spinal cord, which runs from the brain down through the back. It contains threadlike nerves that branch out to every organ and body part.

What are the parts of the brain?

The brain has three main sections: the forebrain, the midbrain, and the hindbrain.

The forebrain is the largest and most complex part of the brain. It consists of the

① Adapted from "Brain and nervous system." Hirsch, L. (2018). https://kidshealth.org

cerebrum—the area with all the folds and grooves—as well as other structures under it.

The cerebrum contains the information that essentially makes you who you are: your intelligence, memory, personality, emotion, speech, and ability to feel and move. Specific areas of the cerebrum are in charge of processing these different types of information. These are called lobes, and there are four of them: the frontal, parietal, temporal, and occipital lobes.

The cerebrum has right and left halves, called hemispheres. They're connected in the middle by a band of nerve fibers (the corpus callosum) that lets them communicate. These halves may look like mirror images of each other, but many scientists believe they have different functions. The left side is considered the logical, analytical, objective side; the right side is thought to be more intuitive, creative, and subjective.

The outer layer of the cerebrum is called the cortex (also known as "gray matter"). Information collected by the five senses comes into the brain to the cortex. This information is then directed to other parts of the nervous system for further processing. For example, when you touch the hot stove, not only does a message go out to move your hand, but one also goes to another part of the brain to help you remember not to do that again.

In the inner part of the forebrain sits the thalamus, hypothalamus, and pituitary gland. The thalamus carries messages from the sensory organs like the eyes, ears, nose, and fingers to the cortex. The hypothalamus controls your pulse, thirst, appetite, sleep patterns, and other processes in your body that happen automatically; it also controls the pituitary gland, which makes the hormones that control growth, metabolism, water and mineral balance, sexual maturity, and response to stress.

The midbrain, underneath the middle of the forebrain, acts as a master coordinator for all the messages going in and out of the brain to the spinal cord.

The hindbrain sits underneath the back end of the cerebrum. It consists of the cerebellum, pons, and medulla. The cerebellum—also called the "little brain" because it looks like a small version of the cerebrum—is responsible for balance, movement, and coordination.

The pons and the medulla, along with the midbrain, are often called the brainstem. The brainstem takes in, sends out, and coordinates the brain's messages. It also controls many of the body's automatic functions, like breathing, heart rate, blood pressure, swallowing, digestion, and blinking.

What are the parts of the nervous system?

The nervous system is made up of the central nervous system and the peripheral nervous system. The brain and the spinal cord are the central nervous system. The nerves that go through the whole body make up the peripheral nervous system.

The brain and the spinal cord are protected by bone: the brain by the bones of the skull, and the spinal cord by a set of ring-shaped bones called vertebrae. They're both cushioned by layers of membranes called meninges and a special fluid called cerebrospinal fluid. This fluid helps protect the nerve tissue, keep it healthy, and remove waste products.

How does the nervous system work?

The basic workings of the nervous system depend a lot on tiny cells called neurons. The brain has billions of them, and they have many specialized jobs. For example, sensory neurons send information from the eyes, ears, nose, tongue, and skin to the brain. Motor neurons carry messages away from the brain to the rest of the body.

All neurons relay information to each other through a complex electrochemical process, making connections that affect the way you think, learn, move, and behave.

Intelligence, learning, and memory

As you grow and learn, messages travel from one neuron to another over and over, creating connections, or pathways, in the brain. It's why driving takes so much concentration when someone first learns it, but later is second nature: the pathway became established.

Memory is another complex function of the brain. The things you've done, learned, and seen are first processed in the cortex. Then, if you sense that this information is important enough to remember permanently, it's passed inward to other regions of the brain (such as the hippocampus and amygdala) for long-term storage and retrieval. As these messages travel through the brain, they too create pathways that serve as the basis of memory.

Movement

Different parts of the cerebrum move different body parts. The left side of the brain controls the movements of the right side of the body, and the right side of the brain controls the movements of the left side of the body. When you press your car's accelerator with your right foot, for example, it's the left side of your brain that sends the message allowing you to do it.

Basic body functions

A part of the peripheral nervous system called the autonomic nervous system controls many of the body processes you almost never need to think about, like breathing, digestion, sweating, and shivering. The autonomic nervous system has two parts: the sympathetic nervous system and the parasympathetic nervous system.

The sympathetic nervous system prepares the body for sudden stress, like if you witness a robbery. When something frightening happens, the sympathetic nervous system makes the heart beat faster so that it sends blood quickly to the different body parts that might need it. It also causes the adrenal glands at the top of the kidneys to release adrenaline, a hormone that helps give extra power to the muscles for a quick getaway. This process is known as the body's "fight or flight" response.

The parasympathetic nervous system does the opposite: it prepares the body for rest. It also helps the digestive tract move along so our bodies can efficiently take in nutrients from the food we eat.

(1,119 words)

Task 1

Read the passage above and answer the following questions.

(1) What does the brain do?

(2) What are the parts of the brain?

(3) What are the parts of the brainstem?

(4) What are the parts of the nervous system?

(5) How does the nervous system work?

Task 2

Please label Figure 7-1 with the medical terms you've learned in Theme reading 1.

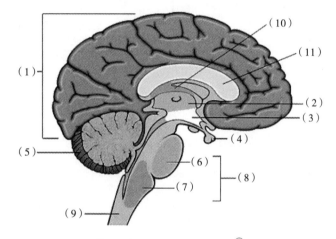

Figure 7-1 Brain structure[①]

(1)	(2)
(3)	(4)
(5)	(6)
(7)	(8)
(9)	(10) basal ganglia
(11)	

① Adapted from *The language of medicine (10th edition)*. Chabner, D-E. (2014). Amsterdam: Saunders/Elsevier.

Task 3

Please fill in the blanks of Figure 7-2 to clarify the main structure of the nervous system. Then, describe the structure on the blanks below the figure.

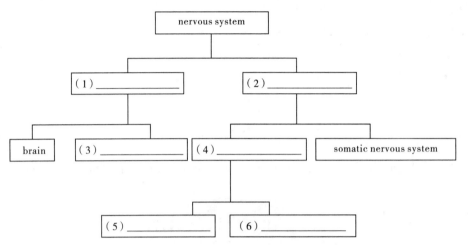

Figure 7-2　Nervous system structure

Your description:

_____

_____

_____

_____

_____

_____

_____

_____

_____

_____

_____

_____

Vocabulary bridge

Study the following terms for common signs, symptoms and diseases related to the nervous system and translate them into Chinese.

Medical terms	Explanation	Chinese translations
Alzheimer's disease	chronic, organic mental disorder that is a progressive form of presenile dementia caused by atrophy of the frontal and occipital lobes of the brain	阿尔茨海默病
epilepsy	disorder affecting the central nervous system that is characterized by recurrent seizures	
palsy	partial or complete loss of motor function; also called paralysis	
cerebral palsy	bilateral, symmetrical, nonprogressive motor dysfunction and partial paralysis, which is usually caused by damage to the cerebrum during gestation or birth trauma but can also be hereditary	
Parkinson disease	progressive, degenerative neurological disorder affecting the portion of the brain responsible for controlling movement	
poliomyelitis	inflammation of the gray matter of the spinal cord caused by a virus, commonly resulting in spinal and muscle deformity and paralysis	
seizure	convulsion or other clinically detectable event caused by a sudden discharge of electrical activity in the brain that may be classified as partial or generalized	

Theme reading 2

Alzheimer's disease[①]

Overview

Alzheimer's disease is a progressive neurologic disorder that causes the brain to shrink (atrophy) and brain cells to die. Alzheimer's disease is the most common cause of dementia—a continuous decline in thinking, behavioral and social skills that affects a person's ability to function independently.

Approximately 5.8 million people in the United States age 65 and older live with Alzheimer's disease. Of those, 80% are 75 years old and older. Out of the approximately 50

---

① Adapted from "Alzheimer's disease" (n. d.). https://www.mayoclinic.org

million people worldwide with dementia, between 60% and 70% are estimated to have Alzheimer's disease.

The early signs of the disease include forgetting recent events or conversations. As the disease progresses, a person with Alzheimer's disease will develop severe memory impairment and lose the ability to carry out everyday tasks.

Medications may temporarily improve or slow progression of symptoms. These treatments can sometimes help people with Alzheimer's disease maximize function and maintain independence for a time. Different programs and services can help support people with Alzheimer's disease and their caregivers.

There is no treatment that cures Alzheimer's disease or alters the disease process in the brain. In advanced stages of the disease, complications from severe loss of brain function—such as dehydration, malnutrition or infection—result in death.

Symptoms

Memory loss is the key symptom of Alzheimer's disease. Early signs include difficulty remembering recent events or conversations. As the disease progresses, memory impairments worsen and other symptoms develop.

At first, a person with Alzheimer's disease may be aware of having difficulty remembering things and organizing thoughts. A family member or friend may be more likely to notice how the symptoms worsen.

Brain changes associated with Alzheimer's disease lead to growing trouble with memory, thinking and reasoning, making judgments and decisions, planning and performing familiar tasks and changes in personality and behavior.

Memory

Everyone has occasional memory lapses, but the memory loss associated with Alzheimer's disease persists and worsens, affecting the ability to function at work or at home.

People with Alzheimer's may repeat statements and questions over and over; forget conversations, appointments and not remember them later; routinely misplace possessions, often putting them in illogical locations; get lost in familiar places; eventually forget the names of family members and everyday objects; and have trouble finding the right words to identify objects, express thoughts or take part in conversations.

Thinking and reasoning

Alzheimer's disease causes difficulty concentrating and thinking, especially about abstract concepts such as numbers.

Multitasking is especially difficult, and it may be challenging to manage finances, balance checkbooks and pay bills on time. Eventually, a person with Alzheimer's may be unable to recognize and deal with numbers.

Making judgments and decisions

Alzheimer's causes a decline in the ability to make reasonable decisions and judgments in everyday situations. For example, a person may make poor or uncharacteristic choices in social interactions or wear clothes that are inappropriate for the weather. It may be more difficult to respond effectively to everyday problems, such as food burning on the stove or unexpected driving situations.

Planning and performing familiar tasks

Once-routine activities that require sequential steps, such as planning and cooking a meal or playing a favorite game, become a struggle as the disease progresses. Eventually, people with advanced Alzheimer's often forget how to perform basic tasks such as dressing and bathing.

Changes in personality and behavior

Brain changes that occur in Alzheimer's disease can affect moods and behaviors. People may suffer depression, apathy, social withdrawal, mood swings, distrust in others, irritability and aggressiveness, changes in sleeping habits, loss of inhibitions, and delusions, such as believing something has been stolen.

Causes

The exact causes of Alzheimer's disease aren't fully understood. But at a basic level, brain proteins fail to function normally, which disrupts the work of brain cells (neurons) and triggers a series of toxic events. Neurons are damaged, lose connections to each other and eventually die.

Scientists believe that for most people, Alzheimer's disease is caused by a combination of genetic, lifestyle and environmental factors that affect the brain over time.

Less than 1% of the time, Alzheimer's is caused by specific genetic changes that virtually guarantee a person will develop the disease. These rare occurrences usually result in disease onset in middle age.

The damage most often starts in the region of the brain that controls memory, but the process begins years before the first symptoms. The loss of neurons spreads in a somewhat predictable pattern to other regions of the brains. By the late stage of the disease, the brain has shrunk significantly.

Researchers trying to understand the cause of Alzheimer's disease are focused on the role of two proteins:

• Plaques. Beta-amyloid is a fragment of a larger protein. When these fragments cluster together, they appear to have a toxic effect on neurons and to disrupt cell-to-cell communication. These clusters form larger deposits called amyloid plaques, which also include other cellular debris.

• Tangles. Tau proteins play a part in a neuron's internal support and transport system to carry nutrients and other essential materials. In Alzheimer's disease, tau proteins change shape and organize themselves into structures called neurofibrillary tangles. The tangles disrupt the transport system and are toxic to cells.

Risk factors

Age

Increasing age is the greatest known risk factor for Alzheimer's disease. Alzheimer's is not a part of normal aging, but as you grow older the likelihood of developing Alzheimer's disease increases.

One study, for example, found that annually there were four new diagnoses per 1,000 people ages 65 to 74, 32 new diagnoses per 1,000 people ages 75 to 84, and 76 new diagnoses per 1,000 people ages 85 and older.

Family history and genetics

Your risk of developing Alzheimer's is somewhat higher if a first-degree relative—your parent or sibling—has the disease. Most genetic mechanisms of Alzheimer's among families remain largely unexplained, and the genetic factors are likely complex.

One better understood genetic factor is a form of the apolipoprotein E gene (APOE). A variation of the gene, APOE e4, increases the risk of Alzheimer's disease. Approximately 25% to 30% of the population carries an APOE e4 allele, but not everyone with this variation of the gene develops the disease.

Scientists have identified rare changes (mutations) in three genes that virtually guarantee a person who inherits one of them will develop Alzheimer's. But these mutations account for less than 1% of people with Alzheimer's disease.

Down syndrome

Many people with Down syndrome develop Alzheimer's disease. This is likely related to having three copies of chromosome 21. Chromosome 21 is the gene involved in the production of the protein that leads to the creation of beta-amyloid. Beta-amyloid fragments can become plaques in the brain. Symptoms tend to appear 10 to 20 years earlier in people with Down syndrome than they do for the general population.

Sex

There appears to be little difference in risk between men and women, but, overall, there are more women with the disease because they generally live longer than men.

Mild cognitive impairment

Mild cognitive impairment (MCI) is a decline in memory or other thinking skills that is greater than normal for a person's age, but the decline doesn't prevent a person from functioning in social or work environments.

People who have MCI have a significant risk of developing dementia. When the primary MCI deficit is memory, the condition is more likely to progress to dementia due to Alzheimer's disease. A diagnosis of MCI encourages a greater focus on healthy lifestyle changes, developing strategies to make up for memory loss and scheduling regular doctor appointments to monitor symptoms.

Head trauma

People who've had a severe head trauma have a greater risk of Alzheimer's disease. Several large studies found that in people age 50 years or older who had a traumatic brain injury (TBI), the risk of dementia and Alzheimer's disease increased. The risk increases in people with more severe and multiple TBIs. Some studies indicate that the risk may be greatest within the first six months to two years after the TBI.

Air pollution

Studies in animals have indicated that air pollution particulates can speed degeneration of the nervous system. Human studies have also found that air pollution exposure—particularly from traffic exhaust and burning wood—is associated with greater dementia risk.

Excessive alcohol consumption

Drinking large amounts of alcohol has long been known to cause brain changes. Several large studies and reviews found that alcohol use disorders were linked to an increased risk of dementia, particularly early-onset dementia.

Poor sleep patterns

Research has shown that poor sleep patterns, such as difficulty falling asleep or staying asleep, are associated with an increased risk of Alzheimer's disease.

Lifestyle and heart health

Research has shown that the same risk factors associated with heart disease also increase the risk of Alzheimer's disease. These include a lack of exercise, obesity, smoking or exposure to secondhand smoke, high blood pressure, high cholesterol, and poorly controlled type 2 diabetes.

These factors can all be modified. Therefore, changing lifestyle habits can to some degree alter your risk. For example, regular exercise and a healthy low-fat diet rich in fruits and vegetables are associated with a decreased risk of developing Alzheimer's disease.

Lifelong learning and social engagement

Studies have found an association between lifelong involvement in mentally and socially stimulating activities and a reduced risk of Alzheimer's disease. Low education levels—less than a high school education—appear to be a risk factor for Alzheimer's disease.

Complications

Memory and language loss, impaired judgment and other cognitive changes caused by Alzheimer's can complicate treatment for other health conditions. A person with Alzheimer's disease may not be able to communicate the experiencing pain, have difficulties to explain symptoms of another illness, and hardly follow a prescribed treatment plan.

As Alzheimer's disease progresses to its last stages, brain changes begin to affect physical functions, such as swallowing, balance, and bowel and bladder control. These effects can increase vulnerability to the following additional health problems:

- inhaling food or liquid into the lungs

- flu, pneumonia and other infections
- falls
- fractures
- bedsores
- malnutrition or dehydration
- constipation or diarrhea
- dental problems such as mouth sores or tooth decay

Prevention

Alzheimer's disease is not a preventable condition. However, a number of lifestyle risk factors for Alzheimer's can be modified. Evidence suggests that changes in diet, exercise and habits—steps to reduce the risk of cardiovascular disease—may also lower your risk of developing Alzheimer's disease and other disorders that cause dementia. Heart-healthy lifestyle choices that may reduce the risk of Alzheimer's include exercising regularly, eating a diet of fresh produce, healthy oils and foods low in saturated fat such as a Mediterranean diet, following treatment guidelines to manage high blood pressure, diabetes and high cholesterol, and asking your doctor for help to quit smoking if you smoke.

Studies have shown that preserved thinking skills later in life and a reduced risk of Alzheimer's disease are associated with participating in social events, reading, dancing, playing board games, creating art, playing an instrument, and other activities that require mental and social engagement.

(1,823 words)

Task 1

Read the passage above and answer the following questions.

(1) What is Alzheimer's disease?

(2) What are the symptoms of Alzheimer's disease?

(3) What do you know about the memory loss of people with Alzheimer's disease?

(4) What are the changes in personality and behavior in patients with Alzheimer's disease?

(5) What are the causes of Alzheimer's disease?

(6) What are the potential risk factors for Alzheimer's disease?

(7) What is the greatest known risk factor for Alzheimer's disease?

(8) What are the complications of Alzheimer's disease?

(9) What can you do to lower the risk of developing Alzheimer's disease?

(10) What heart-healthy lifestyle choices are mentioned in the passage?

Task 2

Read the following paragraph carefully and fill in the blanks with the words from the box.

behavioral	transmit	ranked	cognitive	connections
named	ranges	unpredictable	interferes	dementia

Alzheimer's disease is currently (1)_____ as the seventh leading cause of death in the United States and is the most common cause of (2)_____ among older adults. Dementia is the loss of (3)_____ functioning—thinking, remembering, and reasoning—and (4)_____ abilities to such an extent that it (5)_____ with a person's daily life and activities. Dementia (6)_____ in severity from the mildest stage, when it is just beginning to affect a person's functioning, to the most severe stage, when the person must depend completely on others for help with basic activities of daily living. Alzheimer's disease is (7)_____ after Dr. Alois Alzheimer. In 1906, Dr. Alzheimer noticed changes in the brain tissue of a woman who had died of an unusual mental illness. Her symptoms included memory loss, language problems, and (8)_____ behavior. After she died, he examined her brain and found many abnormal clumps (now called amyloid plaques) and tangled bundles of fibers. These plaques and tangles in the brain are still considered some of the main features of Alzheimer's disease. Another feature is the loss of (9)_____ between neurons in the brain. Neurons (10)_____ messages between different parts of the brain, and from the brain to muscles and organs in the body.

Task 3

Study the boldfaced words in each of the following sentences and make a sentence of your own.
(1) A person with Alzheimer's disease will develop severe memory impairment and lose the ability to **carry out** everyday tasks.

Your sentence: This stable internal environment is necessary for the cells of the body to survive and **carry out** their functions effectively.

(2) The memory loss **associated with** Alzheimer's disease persists and worsens, affecting the ability to function at work or at home.

Your sentence: _____

_____

(3) Scientists believe that for most people, Alzheimer's disease is caused by **a combination of** genetic, lifestyle and environmental factors that affect the brain over time.

Your sentence: _____

_____

(4) Alzheimer's is not a part of normal aging, but as you grow older **the likelihood of** developing Alzheimer's disease increases.

Your sentence: _____

_____

(5) There appears to be little **difference in** risk between men and women, but, overall, there are more women with the disease because they generally live longer than men.

Your sentence: _____

_____

(6) When the primary MCI deficit is memory, the condition is more likely to **progress to** dementia due to Alzheimer's disease.

Your sentence: _____

_____

Task 4

Reorder the following sentences into a reasonable paragraph.

(1) Because of his contributions, he was awarded China's 2008 State Top Scientific and Technological Awards. Only 20 scientists have been bestowed this honor since its foundation in 2000.

(2) After attending the first training course at Beijing Tongren Hospital in 1955, he was nominated to organize a department of neurosurgery in China.

(3) In 1958, after Beijing Xuanwu Hospital was founded, Dr. Wang brought his neurosurgical team to Xuanwu Hospital. Two years later, the Beijing Neurosurgical Institution was founded.

(4) In 1982, after 30 years of hard work, Dr. Wang founded Department of Neurosurgery in Beijing Tiantan Hospital which can treat a full range of neurological disorders from brain tumor to Alzheimer's disease.

(5) Dr. Wang Zhongcheng was born in December 1925 in Shandong Province, China, and obtained his medical education at Medical School of Peking University from 1944 to 1950.

(6) In 1985, he established the *Chinese Journal of Neurosurgery* so that neurosurgery papers no longer had to be published in journals of surgery or neurology.

Correct order: _____ _____ _____ _____ _____ _____

Story sharing

> The following passage[①] is a story about Lauren and Michael. Like many couples, Lauren and Michael have had children, challenges, joys and regrets. But one thing they never planned for, or ever thought about, was the possibility of Alzheimer's wreaking havoc on their family. Please read the story and finish the tasks.

It was only the second time we'd played tennis together when Lauren blurted out, "My husband Michael was just fifty-eight when he died." She had won a fierce point with a put-away volley and her tone sounded matter-of-fact. I froze, taking stock of my partner. Lauren looked mid-sixty, outgoing, attractive, energetic. I had no idea that her husband was dead or why she suddenly felt the urge to talk about him.

"What happened?" I asked, nervous about her response.

"He died from early-onset Alzheimer's." It was two-and-a-half years ago, she said. "I think about him every day."

After the game, we sat and talked for a few minutes. I told her I was a writer and that I'd love to find out more about her personal experience with early-onset Alzheimer's, to share the information with others. My eighty-six-year-old father has dementia too, I mentioned, although its import seemed somehow diminished in light of her loss.

What I didn't say was that I'd remarried only eighteen months earlier and my husband was sixty-one. Although his brain function seems just fine, his father had died from Alzheimer's and his mother had begun developing dementia symptoms before she died. My own father was in the late stage. The scary fact is that every sixty-seven seconds someone in America develops Alzheimer's disease. Lauren's story is all of ours.

The romance

We met for coffee a couple of weeks later and chatted easily about her life and love affair with her husband, and not so easily about his illness and death. "I remember the first time I saw him like it was yesterday," she said. "I was twelve and he was fourteen. It was during recess in the gymnasium. I said, 'Wow! Who's that?'" Three years later, at a New Year's Eve party, he came up and kissed her. "He was the best kisser," she said, smiling and misty-eyed at the memory.

They married when she was twenty. She'd gone to junior college and was an administrative assistant at a big New York City ad agency. He was determined to go to law

---

① Adapted from "The tragedy of early onset Alzheimer's: a friend's story." Araujo, K. (2015). https://betterafter50.com

school, working evenings in a liquor store to pay for it. Six years after graduating from an Ivy, he'd become partner at a firm, specializing in international and corporate law. She was a stay-at-home mom to their four children. They became grandparents and remained close to their own parents. In 1997, Michael left the law firm and opened his own asset management consultancy. Life was good. The couple divided their time between New York and South Florida.

"We had a great friendship and a passion that never died," Lauren said. She pulled out her phone and showed me a couple of photos of her husband. He was, as she had described, tall and handsome. "He was my rock. My best friend and protector."

Strange symptoms

But in late 2004 Lauren noticed that Michael was experiencing some peculiar slips of the tongue. "I thought they were flukes," she said. "He tried to cover them up." He occasionally mispronounced familiar words and asked an awkward question after a friend told them a tragic story. In January 2005 he fumbled for words at a condominium board meeting. "Speech problems—Michael?" Lauren said, still sounding disbelieving. "He'd studied Latin. He had a great gift for language and perfect grammar. I knew something was wrong." He'd been on blood pressure medication since he was twenty-two. Maybe he'd developed a new side effect?

Standing at more than six feet tall, Michael's posture had always been erect. But now Lauren noticed that his neck appeared to be jutting forward. Was this just how men aged? She began watching other men walking down the beach. Their necks seemed fine. Another clue that something was a miss.

In mid-April that year, Michael asked her what her plans were for the next day. "He always listened to where I was going," she said. "I was his focus, even when we had four kids at home." She told him and he nodded. Fifteen seconds later, he asked, "What are you up to tomorrow?"

Because he was still in his fifties, Lauren and Michael didn't rush right away to the doctor. Who thinks of dementia when you still feel like you're in the prime of your life? But by October 2005, they were playing doubles and he couldn't keep track of the tennis score or who was serving.

The diagnosis

They went to see a neurologist. Michael refused some diagnostics but agreed to an MRI and a PET scan, an imaging test that uses a radioactive substance to see how organs and tissues are functioning.

The neurologist's conclusion: clear evidence of neurological degeneration in the lobes, most likely due to Alzheimer's disease.

"Michael never expressed any emotion about the results," Lauren said. "He always said, 'It's not going to affect me. I'm going to live 'til my eighties.'" But the disease progressed at a steady and devastating pace. By the end of 2007 he was forced to close his business.

Lauren grappled with her limited financial knowledge. "I had gone from living with my parents to having Michael take care of me. I didn't know anything about our money, insurance, taxes. That was a huge anxiety."

One of their children had built a successful career in finance and helped Lauren understand her complicated assets. But for the most part, she and Michael kept the illness a secret from other family members and friends. "I told my daughter and my mother," she said, "but few others until 2008 when I called our friends and told everybody." They kept it hidden, she explained, because of the stigma attached to Alzheimer's. "I was embarrassed and ashamed. I didn't want to be put in that category. But I was protecting Michael's dignity too. He was a private, accomplished, confident man. Watching him deteriorate was a terrible thing."

The decline

Lauren cared for him in their home for as long as she could. Michael's speech became disjointed. He refused to shower or change his clothes. He still sat at his desk each day but was unable to function.

By January 2009 it was time to move him to an assisted living residence. Lauren mourned the romance they'd shared, their travel, affection and conversation. "I missed lying next to him in bed," she confided. And while she did sometimes hold Michael in her arms, he never held her back. When she brought him home he went to the bathroom on the rug. He had a seizure in 2009 and Lauren admitted that she wished for his death. By 2011 he'd become aggressive with her. After being admitted to the psychiatric ward of the hospital where they over-sedated him, he became unresponsive. Then he fell and broke his hip. Michael died in a nursing home two weeks later.

It was eight years after the symptoms emerged, precisely the lifespan experts predict for victims of early-onset Alzheimer's.

Advice and resources

Today, 200,000 Americans suffer from the disease, just five percent of all Alzheimer's patients. Yet because Alzheimer's that occurs between the ages of thirty and sixty-five is relatively uncommon and because it is difficult to detect, many suffer for months or even years before diagnosis. There is no cure but there are treatments. Online resources are available. The symptoms often mirror those of other forms of dementia: memory loss, new difficulties with speaking or writing, confusion, to name just a few.

"I still see him coming down the stairs," Lauren said, sounding comforted by the vision. And while she has cleared out his closets, she held onto his favorite navy blazer, loafers, ties and shirt. "I've only had one dream about him these last two years," she said, dabbing her eyes with a napkin. "He kissed me. I felt his lips. But he's gone."

(1,302 words)

Task 1

Read the passage above and write a paragraph to complete it, with the first sentence being provided.

Lauren's best advice to others who may be confronting early-onset Alzheimer's is simple: face it if it's there.

_____

_____

_____

_____

_____

_____

_____

_____

_____

_____

_____

_____

_____

_____

Task 2

Please discuss the following questions in groups.

(1) What was something "off" with Michael Lauren noticed before diagnosis?

(2) Why did Lauren and Michael hide Michael's illness from most family members and friends?

(3) What lessons can you learn from Lauren's role as a wife after diagnosis?

(4) What advice about Alzheimer's disease would you like to give to people at 35 to 65?

Vocabulary checklist

英文	中文
* **nervous** system [ˈnɜːvəs]	神经系统
* digestion [daɪˈdʒestʃən]	消化
* **spinal** cord [ˈspaɪnl]	脊髓
* forebrain [ˈfɔːbreɪn]	前脑
* midbrain [ˈmɪdbreɪn]	中脑
* hindbrain [ˈhaɪndbreɪn]	后脑
* cerebrum [səˈriːbrəm]	大脑
* **frontal** lobe [ˈfrʌntl]	额叶
* **parietal** lobe [pəˈraɪɪt(ə)l]	顶叶
* **temporal** lobe [ˈtempərəl]	颞叶
* **occipital** lobe [ɒkˈsɪpɪtl]	枕叶
corpus callosum [ˈkɔːpəs kəˈləusəm]	胼胝体
* cortex [ˈkɔːteks]	皮质
* thalamus [ˈθæləməs]	丘脑
* hypothalamus [ˌhaɪpəˈθæləməs]	下丘脑
* pituitary gland [pɪˈtjuːɪtəri ɡlænd]	垂体

英文	中文
* hormone [ˈhɔːməʊn]	激素
* metabolism [məˈtæbəlɪzəm]	新陈代谢
* cerebellum [ˌserəˈbeləm]	小脑
* pons [pɒnz]	脑桥
* medulla [meˈdʌlə]	髓质
* brainstem [ˈbreɪnstem]	脑干
* central nervous system	中枢神经系统
* **peripheral** nervous system [pəˈrɪfərəl]	周围神经系统
* vertebrae [ˈvɜːtɪbreɪ]	脊椎(vertebra 的复数)
meninges [məˈnɪndʒiːz]	脑膜;髓膜;脑脊膜(meninx 的复数)
cerebrospinal fluid [ˌserɪbrəʊˈspaɪnəl]	脑脊液
* neuron [ˈnjʊərɒn]	神经元
* **sensory** neuron [ˈsensəri]	感觉神经元
* **motor** neuron [ˈməʊtə(r)]	运动神经元
electrochemical process [ɪˌlektrəʊˈkemɪkəl]	电化过程
hippocampus [ˌhɪpəˈkæmpəs]	海马体
amygdala [əˈmɪgdələ]	杏仁核

英文	中文
* **autonomic** nervous system [ˌɔːtəˈnɒmɪk]	自主神经系统
* **sympathetic** nervous system [ˌsɪmpəˈθetɪk]	交感神经系统
* **parasympathetic** nervous system [ˌpærəˌsɪmpəˈθetɪk]	副交感神经系统
* **adrenal** gland [əˈdriːnl]	肾上腺
adrenaline [əˈdrenəlɪn]	肾上腺素
* digestive tract [daɪˈdʒestɪv trækt]	消化道
* **Alzheimer's** disease [ˈæltshaɪməz]	阿尔茨海默病
* **neurologic** disorder [ˌnjʊərəˈlɒdʒɪkəl]	神经系统疾病
* atrophy [ˈætrəfi]	萎缩
* dementia [dɪˈmenʃə]	痴呆症
memory **impairment** [ɪmˈpeəmənt]	记忆障碍
* medication [ˌmedɪˈkeɪʃn]	药物
* dehydration [ˌdiːhaɪˈdreɪʃn]	脱水
* malnutrition [ˌmælnjuˈtrɪʃn]	营养不良
* symptom [ˈsɪmptəm]	症状
apathy [ˈæpəθi]	冷漠
* delusion [dɪˈluːʒn]	幻觉

英文	中文
* plaque [plɑːk]	斑块
Beta-**amyloid** [ˈæmɪlɔɪd]	β-淀粉样蛋白
amyloid plaque	淀粉样蛋白斑
cellular **debris** [ˈdebriː]	细胞碎片
* tangle [ˈtæŋgl]	缠结
tau protein [tɔː]	tau 蛋白
neurofibrillary tangle [ˌnjʊərəʊfaɪˈbrɪlərɪ]	神经元纤维缠结
sibling [ˈsɪblɪŋ]	兄弟姐妹
apolipoprotein E gene（APOE） [ˌæpəˌlɪpəʊˈprəʊtiːn]	载脂蛋白 E 基因
allele [əˈliːl]	等位基因
* mutation [mjuːˈteɪʃn]	突变
Down **syndrome** [ˈsɪndrəʊm]	唐氏综合征
* chromosome [ˈkrəʊməsəʊm]	染色体
* mild cognitive impairment（MCI）	轻度认知功能障碍
* trauma [ˈtrɔːmə]	创伤
cholesterol [kəˈlestərɒl]	胆固醇
* diabetes [ˌdaɪəˈbiːtiːz]	糖尿病
* bowel [ˈbaʊəl]	肠道

英文	中文
＊bladder [ˈblædə(r)]	膀胱
＊pneumonia [njuːˈməʊniə]	肺炎
＊fracture [ˈfræktʃə(r)]	骨折
bedsore [ˈbedsɔː(r)]	褥疮
＊constipation [ˌkɒnstɪˈpeɪʃn]	便秘
＊diarrhea [ˌdaɪəˈriə]	腹泻
＊**cardiovascular** disease [ˌkɑːdiəʊˈvæskjələ(r)]	心血管疾病
saturated fat [ˈsætʃəreɪtɪd]	饱和脂肪
Mediterranean diet [ˌmedɪtəˈreɪniən]	地中海型饮食
neurologist [njʊəˈrɒlədʒɪst]	神经病学家;神经科专门医师
MRI (Magnetic Resonance Imaging)	磁共振成像
PET Scan (Positron Emission Tomography Scan)	正电子发射层析扫描
deteriorate [dɪˈtɪəriəreɪt]	恶化
disjointed [dɪsˈdʒɔɪntɪd]	不连贯的
seizure [ˈsiːʒə(r)]	(尤指脑病的)突然发作
psychiatric ward [ˌsaɪkiˈætrɪk]	精神科病房
hip [hɪp]	髋

注：＊表示高频医学英语词汇。

Musculoskeletal system

Upon completion of this chapter, you will be able to

❖ name the different types of bones, muscles and joints;

❖ compare the three major types of muscles;

❖ list major pathologic conditions affecting the bones, muscles and joints;

❖ understand information about arthritis;

❖ gather information about common musculoskeletal diseases;

❖ present one common musculoskeletal disease with group members.

Theme reading 1

An introduction to the musculoskeletal system[①]

What are bones and what do they do?

Bones provide support for our bodies and help form our shape. Although they're very light, bones are strong enough to support our entire weight.

Bones also protect the organs in our bodies. The skull protects the brain and forms the shape of the face. The spinal cord, a pathway for messages between the brain and the body, is protected by the backbone, or spinal column. The ribs form a cage that shelters the heart and lungs, and the pelvis helps protect the bladder, part of the intestines, and in women, the reproductive organs.

Bones are made up of a framework of a protein called collagen, with a mineral called calcium phosphate that makes the framework hard and strong. Bones store calcium and release some into the bloodstream when it's needed by other parts of the body. The amounts of

---

① Adapted from "Bones, muscles, and joints" (n.d.). https://kidshealth.org

certain vitamins and minerals that you eat, especially vitamin D and calcium, directly affect how much calcium is stored in the bones.

Bones are made up of two types of bone tissues: compact bone and cancellous bone. Compact bone is the solid, hard outside part of the bone. It looks like ivory and is extremely strong. Holes and channels run through it, carrying blood vessels and nerves. Cancellous bone, which looks like a sponge, is inside compact bone. It is made up of a mesh-like network of tiny pieces of bone called trabeculae. This is where bone marrow is found. In the bone marrow, most of the body's blood cells are made. The bone marrow contains stem cells, which produce the body's red blood cells and platelets, and some types of white blood cells. Red blood cells carry oxygen to the body's tissues, and platelets help with blood clotting when someone has a cut or wound. White blood cells help the body fight infection.

Bones are fastened to other bones by long, fibrous straps called ligaments. Cartilage, a flexible, rubbery substance in our joints, supports bones and protects them where they rub against each other.

How do bones grow?

The bones of kids and young teens are smaller than those of adults and contain "growing zones" called growth plates. These plates consist of multiplying cartilage cells that grow in length, and then change into hard, mineralized bone. These growth plates are easy to spot on an X-ray. Because girls mature at an earlier age than boys, their growth plates change into hard bone at an earlier age.

Bone-building continues throughout life, as a body constantly renews and reshapes the bones' living tissue. Bone contains three types of cells: osteoblasts, osteocytes and osteoclasts. Osteoblasts make new bone and help repair damage. Osteocytes are mature bone cells which help continue new born formation. Osteoclasts break down bone and help to sculpt and shape it.

What are muscles and what do they do?

Muscles pull on the joints, allowing us to move. They also help the body do such things as chewing food and then moving it through the digestive system.

Even when we sit perfectly still, muscles throughout the body are constantly moving. Muscles help the heart beat, the chest rise and fall during breathing, and blood vessels regulate the pressure and flow of blood. When we smile and talk, muscles help us communicate, and when we exercise, they help us stay physically fit and healthy.

Humans have three different kinds of muscle: skeletal muscle, smooth or involuntary muscle, and cardiac muscle.

Skeletal muscle is attached by cord-like tendons to bone, such as in the legs, arms, and face. Skeletal muscles are called striated because they are made up of fibers that have horizontal stripes when viewed under a microscope. These muscles help hold the skeleton together, give the body shape, and help it with everyday movements (known as voluntary muscles because you can control their movement). They can contract (shorten or tighten) quickly and powerfully, but they tire easily.

Smooth or involuntary muscle is also made of fibers, but this type of muscle looks smooth, not striated. We can't consciously control our smooth muscles; rather, they're controlled by the nervous system automatically (which is why they're also called involuntary). Examples of smooth muscles are the walls of the stomach and intestines, which help break up food and move it through the digestive system. Smooth muscle is also found in the walls of blood vessels, where it squeezes the stream of blood flowing through the vessels to help maintain blood pressure. Smooth muscles take longer to contract than skeletal muscles do, but they can stay contracted for a long time because they don't tire easily.

Cardiac muscle is found in the heart. The walls of the heart's chambers are composed almost entirely of muscle fibers. Cardiac muscle is also an involuntary type of muscle. Its rhythmic, powerful contractions force blood out of the heart as it beats.

How do muscles work?

The movements your muscles make are coordinated and controlled by the brain and nervous system. The involuntary muscles are controlled by structures deep within the brain and the upper part of the spinal cord called the brain stem. The voluntary muscles are regulated by the parts of the brain known as the cerebral motor cortex and the cerebellum.

When you decide to move, the motor cortex sends an electrical signal through the spinal cord and peripheral nerves to the muscles, causing them to contract. The motor cortex on the right side of the brain controls the muscles on the left side of the body and vice versa.

The cerebellum coordinates the muscle movements ordered by the motor cortex. Sensors in the muscles and joints send messages back through peripheral nerves to tell the cerebellum and other parts of the brain where and how the arm or leg is moving and what position it's in. This feedback results in smooth, coordinated motion. If you want to lift your arm, your brain sends a message to the muscles in your arm and you move it. When you run, the messages to the brain are more involved, because many muscles have to work in rhythm.

Muscles move body parts by contracting and then relaxing. Muscles can pull bones, but they can't push them back to the original position. So they work in pairs of flexors and extensors. The flexor contracts to bend a limb at a joint. Then, when the movement is completed, the flexor relaxes and the extensor contracts to extend or straighten the limb at the same joint. For example, the biceps muscle, in the front of the upper arm, is a flexor, and the triceps, at the back of the upper arm, is an extensor. When you bend at your elbow, the biceps contracts. Then the biceps relaxes and the triceps contracts to straighten the elbow.

What are joints and what do they do?

Joints are where two bones meet. They make the skeleton flexible—without them, movement would be impossible.

Joints allow our bodies to move in many ways. Some joints open and close like a hinge (such as knees and elbows), whereas others allow for more complicated movement—a shoulder or hip joint, for example, allows for backward, forward, sideways, and rotating movement.

Joints are classified by their range of movement. Immovable or fibrous joints don't move. The dome of the skull, for example, is made of bony plates, which move slightly during birth and then fuse together as the skull finishes growing. Between the edges of these plates are links, or joints, of fibrous tissue. Fibrous joints also hold the teeth in the jawbone. Partially movable or cartilaginous joints move a little. They are linked by cartilage, as in the spine. Each of the vertebrae in the spine moves in relation to the one above and below it, and together these movements give the spine its flexibility. Freely movable or synovial joints move in many directions. The main joints of the body—such as those found at the hip, shoulders, elbows, knees, wrists, and ankles—are freely movable. They are filled with synovial fluid, which acts as a lubricant to help the joints move easily.

Three kinds of freely movable joints play a big part in voluntary movement. Hinge joints allow movement in one direction, as seen in the knees and elbows. Pivot joints allow a rotating or twisting motion, like that of the head moving from side to side. Ball-and-socket joints allow the greatest freedom of movement. The hips and shoulders have this type of joint, in which the round end of a long bone fits into the hollow of another bone.

(1440 words)

Task 1

Read the passage above and answer the following questions.

(1) What are the main functions of bones?

(2) What are the two types of bone tissues? What are their functions respectively?

(3) How do bones grow?

(4) What are the main functions of muscles?

(5) How are involuntary and voluntary muscles controlled by the nervous system respectively?

(6) What are joints and what do they do?

Task 2

Please label Figure 8-1 with the medical terms you've learnt in Theme reading 1 and the terms given below.

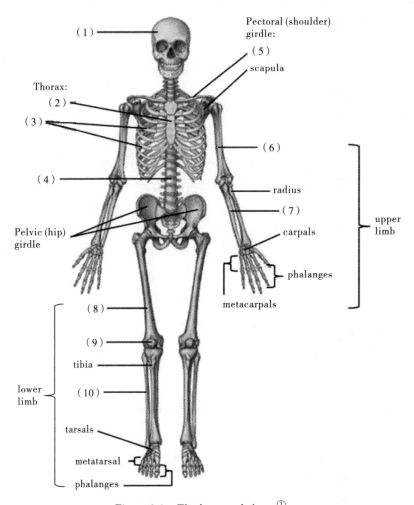

Figure 8-1   The human skeleton[1]

Terms for use

- clavicle: bone linking the scapula and sternum
- femur: the large bone in the upper part of the leg
- fibula: the outer bone of the two bones in the lower part of the leg
- humerus: the bone that extends from the shoulder to the elbow
- patella: a small flat triangular bone in front of and protecting the knee joint
- sternum: the long flat bone which goes from the throat to the bottom of the ribs and to

① Adapted from "The human skeleton" (n. d.). https://spmbiology.blog.onlinetuition.com

which the ribs are attached

· ulna：the inner and longer of the two bones of the human forearm

(1)	(2)
(3)	(4)
(5)	(6)
(7)	(8)
(9)	(10)

Task 3

In Table 8-1, the three major types of muscles of the human body are compared in detail. Please fill in the blanks with words or phrases.

Table 8-1　Comparison of the three major types of muscles①

Pictures of muscle types			
Types of the muscles	(1)	(2)	(3)
Locations	(4)	(5)	(6)
Movement control	(7)	(8)	involuntary

①Adapted from "Muscle atrophy." Knapp, S. (2020). https://biologydictionary.net

Vocabulary bridge

Study the following terms for common signs, symptoms and diseases related to the musculoskeletal system and translate them into Chinese.

Medical terms	Explanation	Chinese translations
muscular dystrophy	group of hereditary diseases characterized by gradual atrophy and weakness of muscle tissue	肌营养不良症
myasthenia gravis	autoimmune neuromuscular disorder characterized by severe muscular weakness and progressive fatigue	
rotator cuff injuries	injuries to the capsule of the shoulder joint, which is reinforced by muscles and tendons	
sprain	trauma to a joint that causes injury to the surrounding ligament, accompanied by pain and disability	
strain	trauma to a muscle from overuse or excessive forcible stretch	
talipes equinovarus	congenital deformity of the foot	
tendinitis	inflammation of a tendon, usually caused by injury or overuse	
torticollis	spasmodic contraction of the neck muscles, causing stiffness and twisting of the neck	
carpal tunnel syndrome (CTS)	pain or numbness resulting from compression of the median nerve within the carpal tunnel (wrist canal through which the flexor tendons and median nerve pass)	
contracture	fibrosis of connective tissue in the skin, fascia, muscle, or joint capsule that prevents normal mobility of the related tissue or joint	
crepitation	grating sound made by movement of bone ends rubbing together, indicating a fracture or joint destruction	
Ewing sarcoma	malignant tumor that develops from bone marrow, usually in long bones or the pelvis	
gout	hereditary metabolic disease that is a form of acute arthritis, characterized by excessive uric acid in the blood and around the joints	
herniated disk	herniation or rupture of the nucleus pulposus (center gelatinous material within an intervertebral disk) between two vertebrae	
osteoporosis	decrease in bone density with an increase in porosity, causing bones to become brittle and increasing the risk of fractures	
Paget disease of bone	skeletal disease affecting elderly people that causes chronic inflammation of bones, resulting in thickening and softening of bones and bowing of long bones	

Medical terms	Explanation	Chinese translations
rheumatoid arthritis (RA)	chronic, systemic inflammatory disease affecting the synovial membranes of multiple joints, eventually resulting in crippling deformities	
subluxation	partial or complete dislocation	
sequestrum	fragment of a necrosed bone that has become separated from surrounding tissue	
ankylosing spondylitis	chronic inflammatory disease of unknown origin that first affects the spine and is characterized by fusion and loss of mobility of two or more vertebrae	
kyphosis	increased curvature of the thoracic region of the vertebral column, leading to a humpback posture	
lordosis	forward curvature of lumbar region of the vertebral column, leading to a swayback posture	
scoliosis	abnormal sideward curvature of the spine to the left or right	
spondylolisthesis	partial forward dislocation of one vertebra over the one below it, most commonly the fifth lumbar vertebra over the first sacral vertebra	

Theme reading 2

Arthritis[①]

Arthritis is a disease that affects your joints (areas where your bones meet and move). Arthritis usually involves inflammation or degeneration (breakdown) of your joints. These changes can cause pain when you use the joint.

Arthritis is most common in the following areas of the body: feet, hands, hips, knees, and lower back.

Joints get cushioned and supported by soft tissues that prevent your bones from rubbing against each other. A connective tissue called articular cartilage plays a key role. It helps your joints move smoothly without friction or pain.

Some joints have a synovial membrane, a padded pocket of fluid that lubricates the joints. Many joints, such as your knees, get supported by tendons and ligaments. Tendons connect muscles to your bones, while ligaments connect bones to other bones.

---

① Adapted from "Arthritis" (n.d.). https://my.clevelandclinic.org

Common types of arthritis

Arthritis is a broad term that describes more than 100 different joint conditions. The most common types of arthritis include osteoarthritis, ankylosing spondylitis, juvenile arthritis (JA), gout, psoriatic arthritis, and rheumatoid arthritis. Osteoarthritis, or "wear and tear" arthritis, develops when joint cartilage breaks down from repeated stress. It's the most common form of arthritis. Ankylosing spondylitis is also called arthritis of the spine (usually your lower back). Juvenile arthritis (JA) is a disorder where the immune system attacks the tissue around joints. JA typically affects children 16 or younger. Gout is a disease that causes hard crystals of uric acid to form in your joints. Psoriatic arthritis is joint inflammation that develops in people with psoriasis (autoimmune disorder that causes skin irritation). Rheumatoid arthritis is a disease that causes the immune system to attack synovial membranes in your joints.

Arthritis is the most common cause of disability in the U.S. About 50 million adults and 300,000 children manage some form of arthritis.

Causes and symptoms

Different types of arthritis have different causes. For instance, gout is the result of too much uric acid in your body. But for other types of arthritis, the exact cause is unknown. You may develop arthritis if you have a family history of arthritis, have a job or play a sport that puts repeated stress on your joints, or have certain autoimmune diseases or viral infections.

Some factors make you more likely to develop arthritis, including age, lifestyle, sex and weight. The risk of arthritis increases as you get older. Smoking or a lack of exercise can increase your risk of arthritis. Most types of arthritis are more common in women. Obesity puts extra strain on your joints, which can lead to arthritis.

Different types of arthritis have different symptoms. They can be mild in some people and severe in others. Joint discomfort might come and go, or it could stay constant. Common symptoms include pain, redness, stiffness, swelling, tenderness and warmth.

Diagnosis and tests

If you think you may have arthritis, see your healthcare provider. The provider will ask about your symptoms and learn how joint pain affects your life. Your provider will perform a physical exam, which may include assessing mobility and range of motion in your joints, checking for areas of tenderness or swelling around your joints, and evaluating your overall health to determine if a different condition could be causing your symptoms.

Imaging exams can help your healthcare provider get a clear picture of your bones, joints and soft tissues. An X-ray, MRI or ultrasound can reveal bone fractures or dislocations that may be causing you joint pain, cartilage breakdown around your joints, muscle, ligament or tendon injuries near your joints, and soft tissue inflammation.

There is no blood test that can directly detect arthritis. But if your healthcare provider suspects gout or rheumatoid arthritis, they may order blood work. It looks for uric acid or inflammatory proteins.

Management and treatment

There's no cure for arthritis, but there are treatments that can help you manage the condition. Your treatment plan will depend on the severity of the arthritis, its symptoms and your overall health.

Conservative (nonsurgical) treatments include medication, physical therapy, and therapeutic injections. Anti-inflammatory and pain medications may help relieve your arthritis symptoms. Some medications, called biologics, target your immune system's inflammatory response. A healthcare provider may recommend biologics for your rheumatoid or psoriatic arthritis. Rehabilitation can help improve strength, range of motion and overall mobility. Therapists can teach you how to adjust your daily activities to lessen arthritic pain. Cortisone shots may help temporarily relieve pain and inflammation in your joints. Arthritis in certain joints, such as your knee, may improve with a treatment called viscosupplementation. It injects lubricant to help joints move smoothly.

Healthcare providers usually only recommend surgery for certain severe cases of arthritis. These are cases that haven't improved with conservative treatments. Surgical options include fusion and joint replacement. Fusion means two or more bones are permanently fused together. It immobilizes a joint and reduces pain caused by movement. Joint replacement means that a damaged, arthritic joint gets replaced with an artificial joint. Joint replacement preserves joint function and movement. Examples include ankle replacement, hip replacement, knee replacement and shoulder replacement.

Prevention and prognosis

You can lower your chances of developing arthritis by avoiding tobacco products, doing low-impact, non-weight bearing exercise, maintaining a healthy body weight, and reducing your risk of joint injuries.

Since there's no cure for arthritis, most people need to manage arthritis for the rest of their lives. Your healthcare provider can help you find the right combination of treatments to reduce symptoms. One of the biggest health risks associated with arthritis is inactivity. If you become sedentary from joint pain, you may face a greater risk for cancer, heart disease, diabetes and other serious conditions.

Changing your routine can make living with arthritis easier. Adjust your activities to lessen joint pain. It may help to work with an occupational therapist (OT). An OT is a healthcare provider who specializes in managing physical challenges like arthritis.

An OT may recommend adaptive equipment, such as grips for opening jars, techniques for doing hobbies, sports or other activities safely, and tips for reducing joint pain during arthritic flare-ups.

Some people find that arthritis feels worse during certain types of weather. Humidity and cold are two common triggers of joint pain.

There are a variety of reasons why this might happen. People tend to be less active in rainy seasons and the wintertime. The cold and damp can also stiffen joints and aggravate arthritis. Other theories suggest that barometric pressure, or the pressure of the air around us, may have some effect on arthritis.

If you find that certain types of weather make your arthritis worse, talk to your healthcare provider about ways to manage your symptoms. Dressing warmly, exercising inside or using heat therapy may help relieve your pain.

(1,119 words)

Task 1

Read the passage above and answer the following questions.

(1) What is arthritis?

(2) What body parts are usually affected in arthritis?

(3) What are the parts of joints?

(4) What are the most common types of arthritis?

(5) What are the risk factors for arthritis?

(6) What are the symptoms of arthritis?

(7) How is arthritis diagnosed?

(8) How can imaging exams help diagnose arthritis?

(9) For what kind of arthritis is a blood test necessary? And why?

(10) How is arthritis treated?

(11) When is surgery needed for arthritis?

(12) Is there anything one can do to prevent arthritis?

(13) What can one do to make living with arthritis easier?

(14) For joint pain triggered by humidity and cold, how could you avoid it?

Task 2

Read the following paragraph carefully and fill in the blanks with the words from the box.

affects	leading	likely	limitations	increase
barrier	demands	determining	excessive	multiple

Arthritis—specifically osteoarthritis (OA), the disease's most common form—has typically been thought of as an age-related problem. Years of wear and tear on joints can cause inflammation, and in turn stiffness and pain. But researchers are now learning that age isn't the (1) _____ factor in osteoarthritis, or OA. "Joint injuries, which can happen in

(2)_____ ways, are a risk factor for OA," says Kelli Allen, PhD, researcher in UNC's Thurston Arthritis Research Center and the Durham Veterans Affairs Medical Center. Major injuries like a torn ACL (前交叉韧带) (3)_____ the risk of OA in the knee joint. At the same time, lots of smaller injuries or (4)_____ joint loading over time can increase risk of OA in joints. All of these instances are common in the military because of the physical (5)_____ and responsibilities of service members. While nearly 1 in 4 Americans have OA, it (6)_____ more than 1 in 3 who have served in the military. Military members older than 40 are twice as (7)_____ to develop arthritis after returning to civilian life, and OA rates in active-duty personnel younger than 20 are 26 percent higher than those of their nonmilitary peers. About half of veterans with arthritis report (8)_____ in their daily activities because of joint symptoms. OA is a (9)_____ cause of immobility among veterans and a major (10)_____ to managing other common health conditions they may have, including cardiovascular disease and diabetes.

Task 3

Study the boldfaced words in each of the following sentences and make a sentence of your own.

(1) One of the biggest **health risks associated with** arthritis is inactivity.

Your sentence: Excess weight is a **health risk associated with** many health problems, including type 2 diabetes, high blood pressure, heart disease and strokes.

(2) Different types of arthritis have different causes. For instance, gout **is the result of** too much uric acid in your body.

Your sentence: _____

(3) Smoking or a lack of exercise can **increase your risk of** arthritis.

Your sentence: _____

(4) You can **lower your chances of** developing arthritis by avoiding tobacco products.

Your sentence: _____

(5) Arthritis is **a disease that affects** your joints (areas where your bones meet and move).

Your sentence: _____

(6) Your treatment plan will **depend on** the severity of the arthritis, its symptoms and your overall health.

Your sentence: _____

Task 4

Reorder the following sentences into a reasonable paragraph.

(1) For instance, arthritis responds very well to acupuncture. When combined with moxa, it can relieve pain and reduce inflammation immediately.

(2) Some acute cases require only a few treatments. While a more chronic, long-term arthritic condition can take months or even years to resolve.

(3) For this reason, it is essential to begin treating this disorder at the earliest stage.

(4) Traditional Chinese treatments reduce pain and inflammation by focusing on eliminating the cause of arthritis.

(5) Needles are placed into points surrounding the painful area, bringing circulation to the area and helping relieve the stagnation that causes pain and swelling.

Correct order: ____ ____ ____ ____ ____

Story sharing

This following story① shares the author's personal experiences of striving to find the best therapy for Mr. B.'s disease, which was previously diagnosed as rheumatoid arthritis by two highly respected clinicians. Please read the story and finish the tasks.

"What have I done?"

The words escaped my mouth like a punctured tire hissing air. I stared at the screen and read it again: *Rheumatoid factor: negative, anti-CCP antibodies: negative.*

For months, I had been caring for Mr. B. and treating what I presumed was severe, deforming rheumatoid arthritis. That was, after all, the condition invoked by his two previous rheumatologists, both of whom are highly respected clinicians in our region. Mr. B. had come to me for care when he felt his tumor necrosis factor inhibitor therapy, which had worked moderately well for him in the past, was waning in efficacy. When we met, I saw what looked like erosive changes in his hands and large rheumatoid nodules just distal to his elbows, and we began the process of trying to find the best therapy for his disease.

But in the months that followed, each change we made—switching to a new medication, adjusting the dose, combining medications—seemed only to worsen his symptoms. His livelihood as a cabinetmaker whose exceptional skill had found him clients among the rich and

---

① Adapted from "Without question." *Jason, L.* (2022). *New England Journal of Medicine*, 386:2456-2457.

famous was being shattered by unending pain and joint swelling. He could not manipulate the tools of his trade, and soon, despite his self-medicating with increasing doses of prednisone, he was walking with crutches and barely leaving his house.

At our most recent visit, I had been shocked by his bulging eyes and flushed, large cheeks protruding from behind his face mask. Though his cushingoid appearance was quite worrisome, even more concerning were the joints in his hands, swollen and purple and exquisitely tender to touch. Seeing all these symptoms, I finally paused in the exam room to wonder: what if I have things all wrong?

A mentor of mine had warned me never to accept the rumor of a diagnosis, but isn't that what I had, in essence, done with Mr. B. when he entered my care? I had not seen all the primary data from years before—his findings on antibody studies and radiographs—so I set to work ordering new tests. As the results trickled in, the diagnosis of rheumatoid arthritis began to seem less and less likely. Gout emerged as a potential alternative explanation for Mr. B.'s symptoms, though I couldn't comprehend how a gout flare would last so many months. By the time we obtained a dual-energy CT scan that all but proved the diagnosis of gout, it was abundantly clear to me that I had failed Mr. B.

There are many ways in which we can fail our patients and many reasons for these failures. We may falter in addressing the emotional needs of a patient even as we provide technically excellent care. We can neglect to offer clear explanations or leave too little time for patients to ask questions, thereby robbing them of their right to engage fully in treatment decisions. Overloaded schedules, lack of knowledge or awareness, stress, burnout, and any number of other obstacles can prevent us from providing ideal care. Yet perhaps the most fundamental way in which we can fail our patients is by not questioning the basic premise of their diagnosis before treating them. It is true that some diagnoses may be self-evident—a hip fracture or a myocardial infarction, for instance—while others, particularly in rheumatology, may be vague, difficult to confirm, and require observation of the patient over time. Nevertheless, keeping an open mind and constantly revisiting the accuracy of a diagnosis is key if we are to best care for our patients and prevent misdiagnosis.

Cognitive diagnostic errors remain extremely common, accounting for up to 70% of all medical errors. The role of these errors in increasing morbidity and mortality is now recognized, and efforts are being made to improve the teaching of critical thinking in medical training and to make physicians aware of cognitive biases and other issues that can increase the risk of diagnostic error.

However, even in the era of electronic medical records, clinicians often meet new patients without having access to the primary data that were used to establish their diagnosis. In such instances, the physician must decide whether or not to accept at face value each part of the reported medical history. For some diagnoses, it may simply be practical and reasonable to trust the records, but physicians promulgate at the patient's peril any previous diagnosis that they accept blindly.

During my rheumatology elective in medical school, our consult team was asked to evaluate a patient with a large, painful knee effusion. The attending physician provided oversight as I aspirated synovial fluid from the knee. I assumed we would await the lab results and then make a diagnosis, but instead the attending led us to the hospital basement, prepared a slide with a few drops of the fluid, and examined the specimen using a polarized light microscope. After scanning the field for a few seconds, he stepped aside so that I could view the abundant monosodium urate crystals. This physician applied the same approach to his evaluation of nearly every piece of clinical data. Together, we looked at radiographs in the dimly lit hospital reading room, we swung by the neuromuscular pathology laboratory to peer at muscle-biopsy slides and learn from the reading pathologist, and so forth. What my attending was seeking to teach me was that in the axiom "trust but verify," verification is the more crucial step.

One would think that such experiences would have solidified that lesson in my consciousness forever, but the siren's call of heuristics and premature closure can be overpowering. When a patient's story or physical exam seems to fit neatly into the diagnosis that we've been handed by a previous clinician, the impulse to go with the flow can be strong. Often, it's only when things don't proceed as expected that we find ourselves asking more probing questions: *Why is the clinical course diverging from the common trajectory? Is this an unusual presentation of the condition I've been treating? Or is it something else altogether?*

In the meantime, the patient suffers until something different is done.

(1,014 words)

Task 1

Read the passage above and write a paragraph to complete it, with the first sentence being provided.

Mr. B. was ultimately started on pegloticase, which has dramatically improved his joint pain and swelling and caused his tophi to shrink significantly.

_____

_____

_____

_____

_____

_____

_____

_____

_____

_____

_____

_____

_____

_____

Task 2

Discuss the following questions in groups.

(1) What lessons can you learn from the author's experience of striving for an accurate diagnosis?

(2) In paragraph seven, the author mentioned obstacles that "prevent us from providing ideal care." What possible obstacles do you think might be there?

(3) How can a doctor refer to previous diagnosis wisely?

(4) As a medical student, what efforts would you make to avoid cognitive diagnostic errors in your future practice?

Vocabulary checklist

英文	中文
* **musculoskeletal** system [ˌmʌskjʊləʊˈskelɪtəl]	肌肉骨骼系统
* spinal cord [ˈspaɪnl kɔːd]	脊髓
* backbone [ˈbækbəʊn]	脊柱
* spinal **column** [ˈkɒləm]	脊柱
* pelvis [ˈpelvɪs]	骨盆，盆腔

英文	中文
* bladder [ˈblædə(r)]	膀胱
* intestine [ɪnˈtestɪn]	肠
* collagen [ˈkɒlədʒən]	胶原,胶原蛋白
compact bone [kəmˈpækt]	密质骨
cancellous bone [ˈkænsələs]	松质骨
trabeculae [trəˈbekjʊliː]	骨小梁(trabecula 的复数)
* platelet [ˈpleɪtlət]	血小板
* clotting [ˈklɒtɪŋ]	凝血
* ligament [ˈlɪɡəmənt]	韧带
* cartilage [ˈkɑːtɪlɪdʒ]	软骨
growth **plate** [pleɪt]	生长板
osteoblast [ˈɒstɪəˌblæst]	成骨细胞
osteocyte [ˈɒstɪəsaɪt]	骨细胞
osteoclast [ˈɒstɪəˌklæst]	破骨细胞
* skeletal muscle [ˈskelətl ˈmʌsl]	骨骼肌
* **involuntary** muscle [ɪnˈvɒləntri]	不随意肌

英文	中文
* **cardiac** muscle [ˈkɑːdiæk]	心肌
* tendon [ˈtendən]	肌腱
striated [ˌstraɪˈeɪtɪd]	有条纹的
* **voluntary** muscle [ˈvɒləntri]	随意肌, 骨骼肌
* **smooth** muscle [ˌsmuːð]	平滑肌
* nervous system	神经系统
* brain **stem** [stem]	脑干
cerebral motor **cortex** [səˈriːbrəl] [ˈkɔːteks]	大脑运动皮层
cerebellum [ˌserəˈbeləm]	小脑
peripheral nerve [pəˈrɪfərəl]	周围神经
* flexor [ˈfleksə(r)]	屈肌
* extensor [ɪkˈstensə(r)]	伸肌
* biceps [ˈbaɪseps]	二头肌
* triceps [ˈtraɪseps]	三头肌
bony plate [ˈbəʊni]	骨板
fibrous joint [ˈfaɪbrəs]	纤维性关节
jawbone [ˈdʒɔːbəʊn]	下颚骨

英文	中文
cartilaginous [ˌkɑːtɪˈlædʒɪnəs]	软骨的
＊ vertebrae [ˈvɜːtɪbreɪ]	椎骨（vertebra 的复数）
synovial fluid [saɪˈnəʊviəl]	滑液
hinge joint [hɪndʒ]	屈戌关节，滑车关节
pivot joint [ˈpɪvət]	枢轴关节
ball-and-socket joint [ˌbɔːlən ˈsɒkɪt]	球窝关节
＊ arthritis [ɑːˈθraɪtɪs]	关节炎
＊ inflammation [ˌɪnfləˈmeɪʃn]	炎症
degeneration [dɪˌdʒenəˈreɪʃn]	退化
articular cartilage [aːˈtɪkjʊlə]	关节软骨
synovial **membrane** [ˈmembreɪn]	滑膜
＊ osteoarthritis [ˌɒstiəʊaːˈθraɪtɪs]	骨关节炎
ankylosing spondylitis [æŋkɪˈləʊzɪŋ ˌspɒndɪˈlaɪtɪs]	强直性脊柱炎
juvenile arthritis [ˈdʒuːvənaɪl]	幼年型关节炎
＊ gout [gaʊt]	痛风
psoriatic arthritis [ˌsɒrɪˈætɪk]	银屑病关节炎

英文	中文
* **rheumatoid** arthritis [ˈruːmətɔɪd]	类风湿性关节炎
psoriasis [səˈraɪəsɪs]	银屑病
autoimmune disorder [ˌɔːtəʊɪˈmjuːn]	自身免疫失调
skin **irritation** [ˌɪrɪˈteɪʃn]	皮肤刺激
stiffness [ˈstɪfnəs]	关节僵直
swelling [ˈswelɪŋ]	肿胀
tenderness [ˈtendənəs]	压痛
bone **fracture** [ˈfræktʃə(r)]	骨折
dislocation [ˌdɪsləˈkeɪʃn]	脱臼
physical therapy	物理治疗
anti-inflammatory [ˌænti ɪnˈflæmətri]	抗炎的
viscosupplementation [ˌvɪskəʊˌsʌplɪmentaʃn]	黏弹性补充疗法
fusion [ˈfjuːʒn]	关节融合术
joint replacement	关节置换术
occupational therapist	职业治疗师
adaptive equipment [əˈdæptɪv ɪˈkwɪpmənt]	自适应设备
flare-up [ˈfleərʌp]	(疾病)突然恶化
rheumatoid factor	类风湿因子

英文	中文
antibody [ˈæntibɒdi]	抗体
rheumatologist [ˌruːməˈtɒlədʒɪst]	风湿病专家
necrosis [neˈkrəʊsɪs]	坏死
nodule [ˈnɒdjuːl]	结节
prednisone [ˈprednɪsəʊn]	泼尼松
myocardial infarction [ˌmaɪəʊˈkɑːdiəl ɪnˈfɑːkʃn]	心肌梗死
rheumatology [ˌruːməˈtɒlədʒi]	风湿病学
morbidity [mɔːˈbɪdəti]	发病率
effusion [ɪˈfjuːʒn]	渗出
neuromuscular pathology [ˌnjʊərəʊˈmʌskjʊlə]	神经肌肉病理学
biopsy [ˈbaɪɒpsi]	活检
* pathologist [pəˈθɒlədʒɪst]	病理学家,病理学医生

注：＊表示高频医学英语词汇。